NEUROSCIENCE RESEARCH PROGRESS

NERVE SHEATH TUMORS

SIGNS, SYMPTOMS AND TREATMENT

NEUROSCIENCE RESEARCH PROGRESS

Additional books and e-books in this series can be found on Nova's website under the Series tab.

RARE DISORDERS RESEARCH PROGRESS

Additional books and e-books in this series can be found on Nova's website under the Series tab.

NEUROSCIENCE RESEARCH PROGRESS

NERVE SHEATH TUMORS

SIGNS, SYMPTOMS AND TREATMENT

RICHARD A. PRAYSON, MD, MED
EDITOR

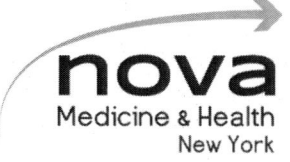

Copyright © 2020 by Nova Science Publishers, Inc.

All rights reserved. No part of this book may be reproduced, stored in a retrieval system or transmitted in any form or by any means: electronic, electrostatic, magnetic, tape, mechanical photocopying, recording or otherwise without the written permission of the Publisher.

We have partnered with Copyright Clearance Center to make it easy for you to obtain permissions to reuse content from this publication. Simply navigate to this publication's page on Nova's website and locate the "Get Permission" button below the title description. This button is linked directly to the title's permission page on copyright.com. Alternatively, you can visit copyright.com and search by title, ISBN, or ISSN.

For further questions about using the service on copyright.com, please contact:
Copyright Clearance Center
Phone: +1-(978) 750-8400   Fax: +1-(978) 750-4470   E-mail: info@copyright.com.

NOTICE TO THE READER

The Publisher has taken reasonable care in the preparation of this book, but makes no expressed or implied warranty of any kind and assumes no responsibility for any errors or omissions. No liability is assumed for incidental or consequential damages in connection with or arising out of information contained in this book. The Publisher shall not be liable for any special, consequential, or exemplary damages resulting, in whole or in part, from the readers' use of, or reliance upon, this material. Any parts of this book based on government reports are so indicated and copyright is claimed for those parts to the extent applicable to compilations of such works.

Independent verification should be sought for any data, advice or recommendations contained in this book. In addition, no responsibility is assumed by the Publisher for any injury and/or damage to persons or property arising from any methods, products, instructions, ideas or otherwise contained in this publication.

This publication is designed to provide accurate and authoritative information with regard to the subject matter covered herein. It is sold with the clear understanding that the Publisher is not engaged in rendering legal or any other professional services. If legal or any other expert assistance is required, the services of a competent person should be sought. FROM A DECLARATION OF PARTICIPANTS JOINTLY ADOPTED BY A COMMITTEE OF THE AMERICAN BAR ASSOCIATION AND A COMMITTEE OF PUBLISHERS.

Additional color graphics may be available in the e-book version of this book.

Library of Congress Cataloging-in-Publication Data

Names: Prayson, Richard A., editor.
Title: Nerve sheath tumors : signs, symptoms and treatment / [edited by
   Richard A. Prayson].
Description: New York : Nova Science Publishers, Inc., [2020] | Series:
   Neuroscience research progress, rare disorders research progress |
   Includes bibliographical references and index. |
Identifiers: LCCN 2020001386 (print) | LCCN 2020001387 (ebook) | ISBN
   9781536173666 (paperback) | ISBN 9781536173673 (adobe pdf)
Subjects: LCSH: Nerves, Peripheral--Tumors. | Myelin sheath--Diseases. |
   Nervous system--Cancer.
Classification: LCC RC280.N4 N465 2020 (print) | LCC RC280.N4 (ebook) |
   DDC 616.99/48--dc23
LC record available at https://lccn.loc.gov/2020001386
LC ebook record available at https://lccn.loc.gov/2020001387

Published by Nova Science Publishers, Inc. † New York

CONTENTS

Preface vii

Chapter 1 Epithelioid Malignant Peripheral Nerve
Sheath Tumors 1
Emad Ababneh and Richard A. Prayson

Chapter 2 Colonic Perineurioma: A Review
of Clinicopathologic Features 21
Lanisha D. Fuller and Richard A. Prayson

Chapter 3 Peripheral Nerve Sheath Tumors
of the Oral Cavity and Jaw 35
Bryan B. Hair and Richard A. Prayson

Chapter 4 Clinicopathologic Features of Salivary Gland
Peripheral Nerve Sheath Tumors 83
Brigid E. Prayson and Richard A. Prayson

Chapter 5 Melanotic Schwannomas:
A Clinicopathologic Review 101
David Sin and Richard A. Prayson

Editor's Contact Information 123

Index 125

Preface

There are a variety of tumors that can arise from various compartments and cellular components of peripheral nerves throughout the body. These peripheral nerve sheath tumors run the gamut from benign, fairly commonly encountered neoplasms such as schwannomas and neurofibromas to rarer, low grade neoplasms and variants such as perineuriomas, mucosal neuromas, palisaded encapsulated neuromas, granular cell tumors and nerve sheath myxomas to malignant neoplasms, so-called malignant peripheral nerve sheath tumors. They are generally classified as soft tissue neoplasms but they differ from most other tumors in this general grouping in a number of ways.

Many of them are associated with genetic disorders or hereditary tumor syndromes and the majority of malignant peripheral nerve sheath tumors arise from a benign precursor tumor, neurofibroma. Their precise diagnosis and classification necessitates careful correlation with clinical and surgical data along with attention to histologic and immunohistochemical features. This text is comprised of a collection of chapters reviewing some of the myriad aspects of this group of neoplasms and includes discussions of the epithelioid variant of malignant peripheral nerve sheaths, perineuriomas arising in the colon, peripheral nerve sheath tumors arising in the oral cavity, jaw and salivary gland regions of the head and neck, and the melanotic variant of schwannoma.

Chapter 1 - Malignant peripheral nerve sheath tumors (MPNSTs) are sarcomas that display differentiation features toward one of the various elements of the nerve sheath. Their diagnosis is one of the most elusive to make in soft tissue pathology due to heterogeneous morphological, histochemical and molecular profiles. Although epithelioid MPNST is considered one morphological variant of these tumors, recent studies revealed that this variant differs substantially from conventional MPNSTs in its clinical, morphological and ultrastructural features. It occurs less frequently in association with neurofibromatosis 1 and more frequently associated with loss of expression of SMARCB1/INI, raising the possibility of an association with schwannomatosis and germline SMARCB1 mutations. They have a wide age of presentation, with most tumors arising on the trunk and showing multinodular growth of large polygonal cells with vesicular chromatin pattern and prominent nucleoli. They are aggressive tumors with at least half the cases showing distant metastasis. In this chapter, the authors will discuss this variant of MPNSTs in detail, reviewing the clinical, pathological and prognostic features with an emphasis on their differential diagnosis and the current available repertoire to make this diagnosis.

Chapter 2 - Perineuriomas are benign neoplasms of the peripheral nerve sheath that are comprised entirely of perineurial cells. These tumors may arise within the intraneural compartment, formerly known as localized hypertrophic neuropathy, or in the soft tissue compartment, formerly known as storiform perineural fibroma. Soft tissue perineuriomas are usually found in the subcutis of extremities and the trunk. Infrequently however, they occur in the gastrointestinal tract, especially in the distal colon. Colonic perineuriomas typically present as small mucosal polyps and are discovered incidentally during screening colonoscopy. Histologically, they are marked by a proliferation of elongated perineurial cells growing in fascicles or bundles that separate the crypts. Perineurial cells are epithelial membrane antigen (EMA), claudin-1 and glucose transporter-1 (GLUT1) positive while negative for S-100 protein, which allows their distinction from other peripheral nerve sheath tumors. They are negative for muscle markers and c-KIT which allows distinction from more common spindle cell neoplasms encountered in the gastrointestinal tract. Differential diagnostic considerations include other nerve sheath tumors as well as leiomyoma and gastrointestinal stromal tumor (GIST).

Chapter 3 - Peripheral nerve sheath tumors of the oral cavity and jaw are rare entities with limited discussion in the literature. There are both benign and malignant tumor subtypes, and although they all derive from nerves or other cells of the neural sheath, their histology, clinical behavior, and preferred treatment strategies are distinct. The following subtypes are included in this chapter: schwannoma, neurofibroma, palisaded encapsulated neuroma, perineurioma, mucosal neuroma, nerve sheath myxoma, granular cell tumor, and malignant peripheral nerve sheath tumor. Traumatic neuroma, though not a true neoplasm, is also included. These neoplasms can occur at disparate locations within the oral cavity such as the submandibular triangle, mandible, palate, lips, oral mucosa, and tongue. Many features are thought to be similar to peripheral nerve sheath tumors of other primary locations, though there are important differences. The differential diagnosis is also distinct for lesions encountered in the oral cavity. Some of the aforementioned tumor types are associated with syndromes such as neurofibromatosis type 1 and multiple endocrine neoplasia type IIB, and there are clinically relevant distinctions between patients with syndromic rather than sporadic tumors. This chapter will consolidate the authors' understanding of this uncommon yet clinically significant tumor category as it relates to epidemiology, tumor etiology, clinical presentation, histopathological characteristics, diagnosis, treatment, and patient outcomes.

Chapter 4 - Salivary gland peripheral nerve sheath tumors are relatively rare neoplasms and their diagnosis is usually not expected preoperatively. Most of the literature focused on the three main tumors in this grouping (schwannomas, neurofibromas, and malignant peripheral nerve sheath tumors) consists of case reports and small series. An association of neurofibromas and plexiform neurofibromas with Neurofibromatosis type I is well documented. The benign tumors (schwannomas and neurofibromas) typically present as slow growing, painless, mobile masses. Malignant peripheral nerve sheath tumors may be painful or non painful masses that often are associated with sudden increased growth. The tumors morphologically resemble their counterparts in other regions of the body. This chapter will review the literature on these three tumor types arising in salivary gland tissue and summarize the clinicopathologic features of these neoplasms.

Chapter 5 - Melanotic schwannomas are relatively rare tumors of the peripheral nervous system. The tumor is well known to be associated with Carney's complex, an autosomal dominant hereditary tumor disorder, additionally marked by lentiginous pigmentation, Cushing's syndrome and myxomas of the heart, skin and breast. Tumors may present at any age and have been documented to arise throughout the body but with a predilection for the spinal nerves. Histopathologically, tumors are marked by spindled to epithelioid cells which contain neuromelanin pigment. A subset of tumors also show evidence of psammoma body formation. Although most tumors behave in a benign fashion, a subset of tumors, unlike conventional schwannoma, can follow a malignant course. Differential diagnostic considerations include other pigmented peripheral nerve sheath tumors, melanocytomas, melanomas, and clear cell sarcomas of soft tissue. This chapter will review the clinicopathologic features of these nerve sheath tumors including discussion of differential diagnosis.

In: Nerve Sheath Tumors
Editor: Richard A. Prayson

ISBN: 978-1-53617-366-6
© 2020 Nova Science Publishers, Inc.

Chapter 1

EPITHELIOID MALIGNANT PERIPHERAL NERVE SHEATH TUMORS

Emad Ababneh, MD *and Richard A. Prayson*, MD, MEd*
Department of Anatomic Pathology, Cleveland Clinic,
Cleveland, Ohio, US

ABSTRACT

Malignant peripheral nerve sheath tumors (MPNSTs) are sarcomas that display differentiation features toward one of the various elements of the nerve sheath. Their diagnosis is one of the most elusive to make in soft tissue pathology due to heterogeneous morphological, histochemical and molecular profiles. Although epithelioid MPNST is considered one morphological variant of these tumors, recent studies revealed that this variant differs substantially from conventional MPNSTs in its clinical, morphological and ultrastructural features. It occurs less frequently in association with neurofibromatosis 1 and more frequently associated with loss of expression of SMARCB1/INI, raising the possibility of an association with schwannomatosis and germline SMARCB1 mutations.

---

* Corresponding Author's Email: praysor@ccf.org; Fax: 216-445-6967.

They have a wide age of presentation, with most tumors arising on the trunk and showing multinodular growth of large polygonal cells with vesicular chromatin pattern and prominent nucleoli. They are aggressive tumors with at least half the cases showing distant metastasis. In this chapter, we will discuss this variant of MPNSTs in detail, reviewing the clinical, pathological and prognostic features with an emphasis on their differential diagnosis and the current available repertoire to make this diagnosis.

INTRODUCTION

Malignant peripheral nerve sheath tumors (MPNSTs) are a varied group of tumors due to their origin from various elements of the nerve sheath. Accordingly, they vary in morphology in light of this variable differentiation. Their diagnosis is an elusive one to make, given the lack of specific morphology or biomarkers. This is especially true for epithelioid malignant nerve sheath tumors (eMPNSTs), a rare and peculiar variant of MPNST.

This variant was first described in a case report by McCormack et al. in 1954 titled "Malignant epithelioid neurilemoma" [1]. In this case report, the authors proposed a simple classification for the different malignant schwannomas (currently known as MPNST) they observed based on the morphology of their constituent cells. They divided them into three types: a pure spindle cell variant, an epithelioid variant, and a neuroepithelial, rosette-forming variant [1]. Interestingly, they made a distinction between conventional (spindle cell) MPNSTs and eMPNSTs, and noted a greater association of the former with neurofibromatosis type 1 (NF1) syndrome (von Recklinghausen's disease) [1]. Despite the numerous case reports and series describing features of eMPNSTs since that time, standardized diagnostic findings and criteria are still lacking. One added layer of challenge is the morphological and immunohistochemical overlap with various other tumors, especially malignant melanoma. In the current surgical pathology practice, the diagnosis of MPNSTs, in general, is considered where an association with a nerve or a benign nerve sheath tumor can be demonstrated, especially in patients with known NF1 syndrome [2-4]. The focus of this chapter is to provide an overview of eMPNSTs, demonstrating their main clinical and pathologic features, as well as provide a concise summary of their main differential diagnoses and practical features to aid in making the distinction.

CLINICAL FEATURES

Epithelioid MPNST is an extremely rare subtype of MPNST. While MPNSTs may represent around 5 - 10% of all soft tissue sarcomas, eMPNSTs represent around 5% of MPNSTs in general [3-6]. They have similar epidemiological and clinical features to conventional MPNSTs [3-6]. They show similar distribution among both sexes. They most commonly arise in adults in their third and fourth decades; nevertheless, cases in children and geriatric patients have been reported [3, 4, 7, 8]. The extremities (mainly lower extremities) are more commonly affected, followed by the trunk and head/neck, but a wide site distribution has been also observed [3, 8-10]. Most patients present with a slowly enlarging mass. Pain has been described in only a subset of patients [3, 6]. Many cases arise from a major nerve or nerve plexuses [3-6]. They differ from conventional MPNSTs in their infrequent association with neurofibromatosis and higher incidence of originating from a preexisting schwannoma [1, 3].

Radiographs are frequently normal. Magnetic resonance imaging (MRI) is the current imaging modality of choice to diagnose peripheral nerve sheath tumors (PNSTs) in general, and this applies to eMPNSTs too [11].

The radiologic diagnosis of eMPNSTs, similar to all PNSTs, often rests on the finding of a fusiform-shape mass with tapered ends, especially if the mass arises from a site of a known nerve [11]. They tend to be heterogeneously enhancing, especially if necrosis is present [11]. Histopathologic examination is required to confirm the diagnosis, as the radiologic features of malignancy are not very reliable and show overlap with benign PNSTs [11].

PATHOLOGY

Grossly, these tumors look similar to their conventional counterparts and are frequently associated with an identified nerve trunk or plexus [3-9, 12]. They have a wide range of sizes from less than a centimeter to more than 20 cm [3-6, 12]; cutaneous cases show ranges on the lower end of the spectrum, possibly due to early diagnosis [3, 6, 12].

Tumors may be solid or cystic, firm, lobulated, tan, and have a fleshy cut surfaces. Grossly apparent hemorrhage and necrosis are frequent occurences [3-6, 12].

On histologic examination, eMPNSTs classically demosntrate a vaguely multinodular growth pattern of large epithelioid, polygonal cells arranged in nests or cords (Figure 1) [3-9, 12, 13].

The cells have moderate-to-abundant, amphophilic to eosinophilic cytoplasm surrounding a large nucleus with vesicular chromatin and a prominent basophilic nucleolus (described by some as "melanoma-like") (Figure 2) [3-6, 12].

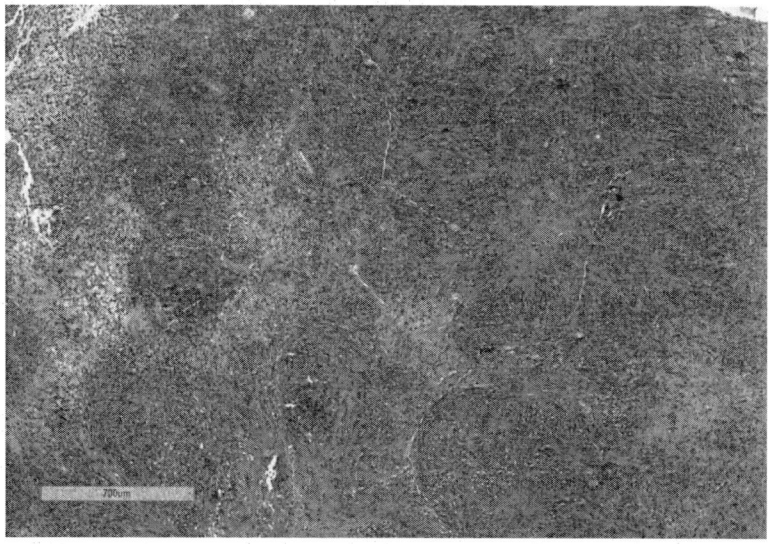

Figure 1. Epithelioid MPNSTs show multinodular proliferation of epithelioid cells with high nuclear-to-cytoplasmic ratios (hematoxylin and eosin, original magnification 30X).

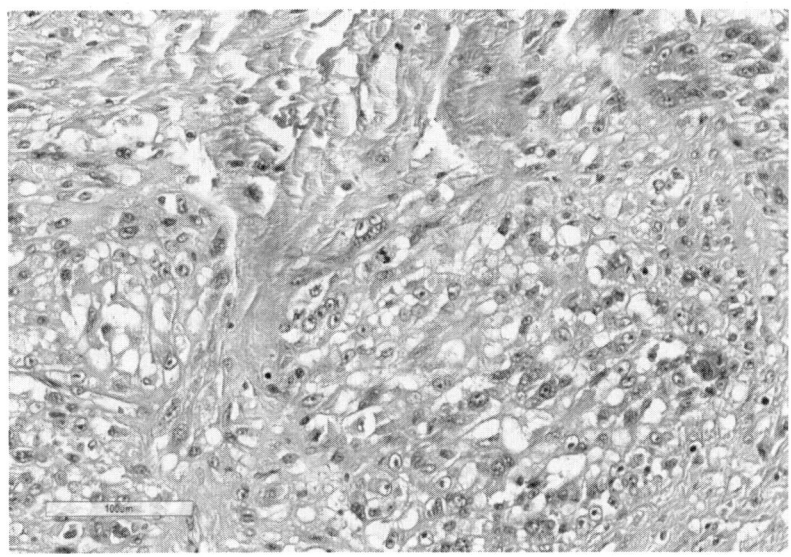

Figure 2. The cells in epithelioid MPNSTs show moderate to severe atypia. They show large nuclei, vesicular chromatin, and prominent nucleoli. Mitotic figures are common finding (hematoxylin and eosin, original magnification 200X).

The cells are fairly uniform but show moderate to severe atypia [3-6]. In the rare occasion of cases showing milder atypia, the atypia and pleomorphism should, at a minimum, be more than would be expected for an epithelioid schwannoma (discussed later) [3, 14, 15]. The cells of eMPNSTs sit in a myxoid and/or fibrous stroma which is often prominent and separates the cells into nests and cords (Figures 3 and 4) [3-6, 12]. Most tumors are well-circumscribed and demonstrate an expansile growth pattern [3-6]. Rarely, tumors are encapsulated. Mitotic figures are present in most cases, and can range from 1 up to 40-50 /10 high power fields (HPF) (Figure 2) [3, 5, 6]. Atypical mitoses can be seen, but they are not a common finding and not necessary for the diagnosis [3]. Necrosis and hemorrhage is a common finding [3-6], and although necrosis is part of the World Health Organization (WHO) grading of sarcomas, its prognostic significance in eMPNSTs is questionable [16, 17]. Tumors arising in association with a schwannoma are not an uncommon finding [3], and schwannomatous areas, whether conventional or epithelioid, might be morphologically evident.

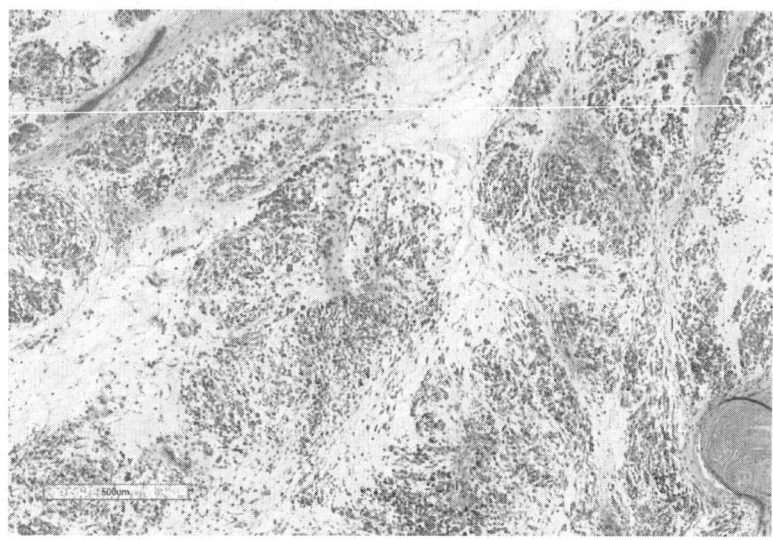

Figure 3. The stroma in epithelioid MPNSTs can be predominantly myxoid (hematoxylin and eosin, original magnification 30X).

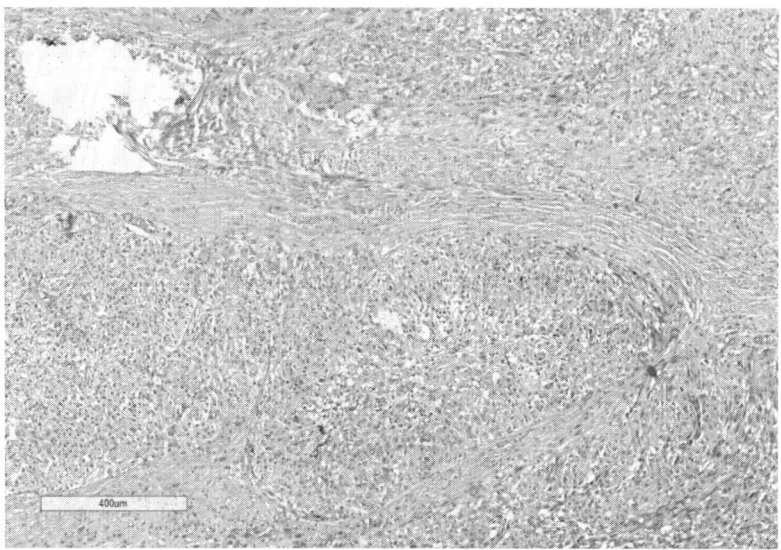

Figure 4. In many cases of epithelioid MPNSTs, the cells show moderate amount of eosinophilic-to- amphophilic cytoplasm. The stroma in this case is predominantly fibrous (hematoxylin and eosin, original magnification 50X).

Other rare morphologies described in the literature include rhabdoid cells, clear cell morphology, perivascular whorling, presence of multinuclear giant cells, and heterologous differentiation with bone or cartilage [3]. S-100 protein expression is the most consistent immunohistochemical feature, which is diffusely positive in virtually all cases (Figure 5) [3, 5, 6]. This feature is one of the major differences in staining patterns compared to conventional MPNSTs, which are mostly negative or focally positive at best [18].

Other reported positive markers in a subset of eMPNSTs are epithelial membrane antigen (EMA) and glial fibrillary acidic protein (GFAP), and their expression is heterogeneous, with both focal and diffuse staining patterns demonstrated [3]. Cytokeratin and HMB45 immunostaining are essentially negative in most cases [3, 5], but some reports rarely describe focal positivity with both markers [2, 6]. Other notable markers, like smooth muscle actin (SMA), desmin, melan A, myogenin and CD31, are reported to be consistently negative [3, 5, 6]. The loss of H3K27 trimethylation (H3K27me3), which is present in about 50% of conventional MPNSTs [19, 20], is not a feature of eMPNSTs, as it is retained in virtually all cases studied in the literature [19, 20].

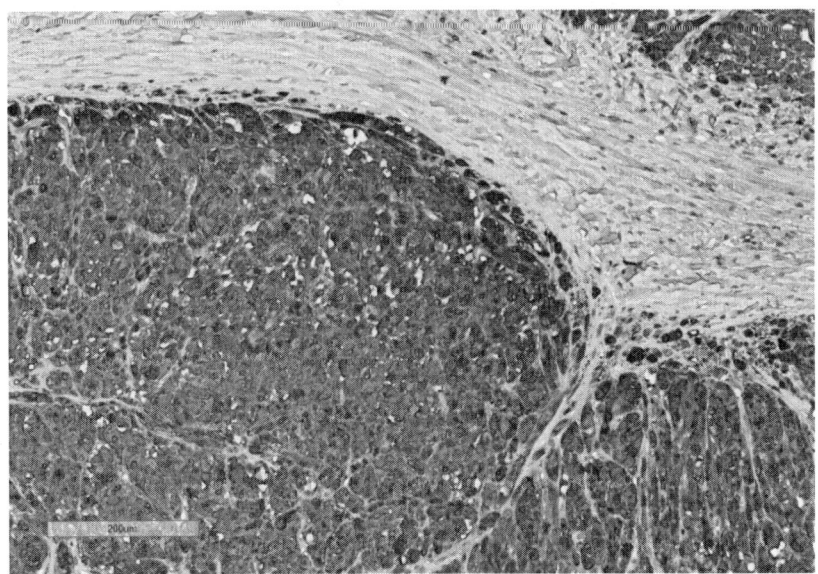

Figure 5. S-100 protein immunostain is diffusely positive in virtually all cases of epithelioid MPNSTs (original magnification 100X).

SMARCB1 (also known as INI-1) is a member of the SWI/SNF chromatin remodeling complex and is involved in regulation of gene expression via epigenetic modification of transcription [21, 22]. It functions mainly as a tumor suppressor gene [21, 22]. Inactivation of SMARCB1, and subsequently the loss of its protein expression by immunohistochemistry, has been demonstrated in many tumors and the list of these tumors is continuously expanding [13, 21-25]. The majority of eMPNSTs (around 70%) show loss of SMARCB1 expression (Figure 6) [21].

Next-generation sequencing studies have detected a high rate of SMARCB1 inactivation [21], a finding that supports the hypothesis that SMARCB1 inactivation plays a major role, and is probably essential for the development of these tumors [21]. Other than this promising understanding of the role of SMARCB1 inactivation, The genomic landscape of eMPNSTs is yet to be defined [21].

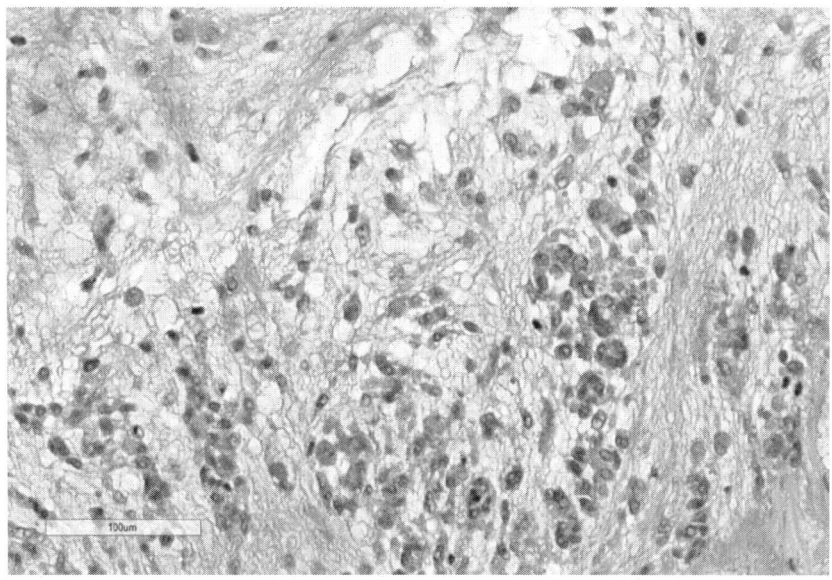

Figure 6. Majority of epithelioid MPNSTs show loss of SMARCB1/INI-1 expression using immunohistochemistry. SMARCB1/INI-1 nuclear expression is retained in normal cells and reactive infiltrating lymphocytes are showing in the background retaining the expression of SMARCB1/INI-1 and serve as an internal control (original magnification 200X).

The role of genetic keydrivers known to be associated with conventional MPNSTs, namely NF1 and PRC2, is poorly understood [21, 26, 27].

DIFFERENTIAL DIAGNOSIS

From the discussion above, one can notice that the not-very specific morphology of eMPNSTs, marked by a nodular proliferation of epithelioid cells combined with a nonspecific staining pattern, makes for a difficult diagnosis because of a potential resemblance to other tumors. The two main challenging and impactful differential diagnoses are epithelioid schwannomas and malignant melanoma.

Epithelioid schwannomas (ESCW) are a rare variant of schwannoma, which most commonly present as uninodular, encapsulated, superficial lesions [14, 15, 28]. They virtually always show clusters of epithelioid cells with a variable degree of cellularity from case to case [14, 15, 28]. Differentiating them from eMPNSTs is important, as they are benign with no risk of metastasis. Making the distinction, though, is challenging, given that the distinction is dependent on the morphologic threshold of atypia [3, 14, 15, 28]. ESCWs also share the immunohistochemical staining pattern with eMPNSTs, as they are diffusely positive for S-100 and large subset of them show loss of SMARCB1 expression [3, 15, 21, 24, 28]. Atypical features, such as large hyperchromatic nuclei, prominent nucleoli, and high mitotic count can be present in ESCW (Figure 7) [15]. These atypical features do not correlate with any prognostic significance [15]. Features that can help differentiate between eMPNST and ESCW are: (A) moderate to severe atypia (as mild atypia can happen in ESCW), defined mainly as large irregular nuclei with vesicular chromatin and prominent nucleoli; (B) the presence of necrosis and/or atypical mitoses, as these should not be present in ESCWs; and (C) the presence of other features of schwannoma in general, such as encapsulation, lymphoid aggregates (Figure 8), nuclear palisading, and perivascular hyalinization, which are variably present and are not as diagnostically useful as (A) and (B) [3, 14, 15, 28].

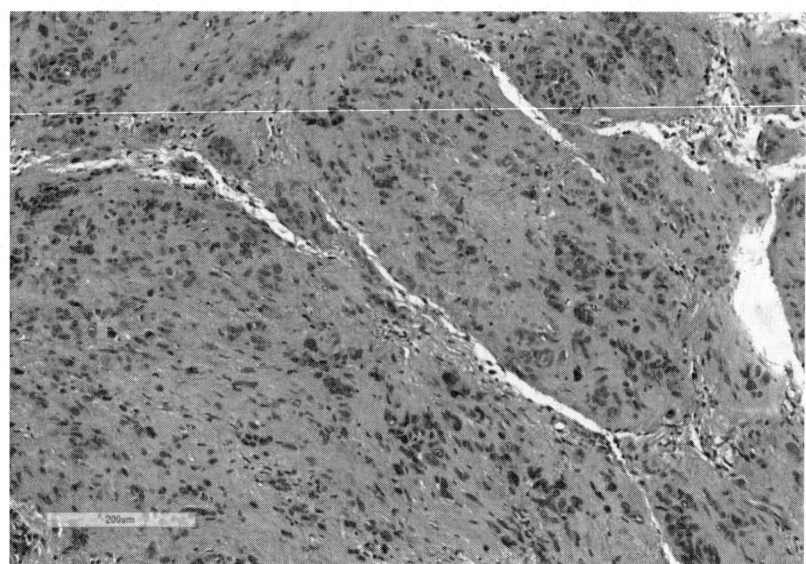

Figure 7. While epithelioid schwannomas can show some degree of atypia, this atypia is mild and should be focal. This finding has no prognostic significance (hematoxylin and eosin, original magnification 100X).

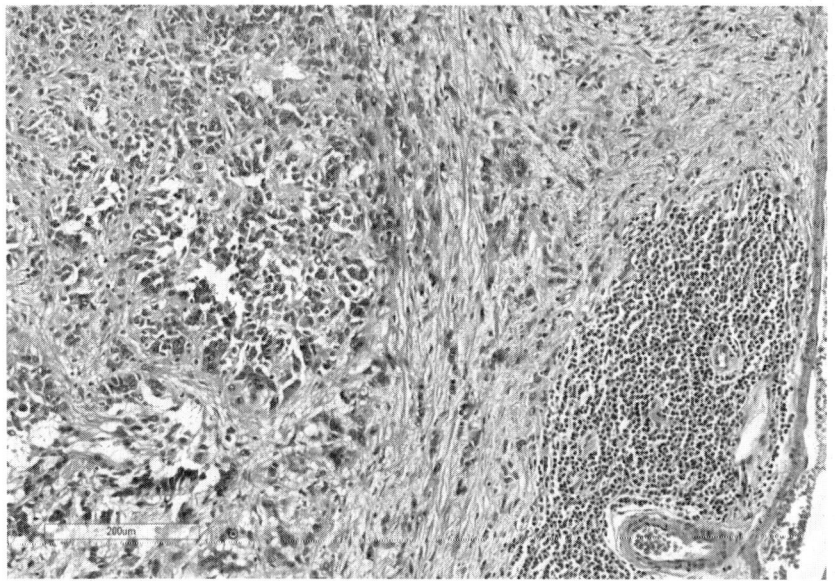

Figure 8. Epithelioid schwannomas show proliferation of epithelioid cells, usually with no-to-minimal atypia. Lymphoid aggregates are commonly found at the periphery of schwannomas (hematoxylin and eosin, original magnification 100X).

Malignant melanomas are another main diagnostic consideration, as they can occur at any site and have a variable morphological spectrum that can overlap with eMPNSTs. On the one hand, many melanoma cases can be straightforward to differentiate from eMPNSTs by the virtue of prior history, a junctional/epidermal component, predominantly spindle cell morphology, and the presence of significant melanin pigment. On the other hand, amelanotic cases of melanoma that show a predominantly nested epithelioid morphology with no apparent epidermal component can pose a challenge (Figure 9), especially since they are usually diffusely positive for S-100 protein [3, 29, 30]. Melanomas usually show a higher degree of pleomorphism and atypia. Myxoid stroma, which is common in eMPNSTs, is a rare occurrence in melanomas, and SMARCB1 (INI-1), which is lost in the majority of eMPNSTs, is retained in the majority, if not all, melanomas [23].

Also, more specific melanocytic markers, melan-A and HMB-45, are invariably negative in eMPNSTs (Figure 10) [3, 5, 6, 29].

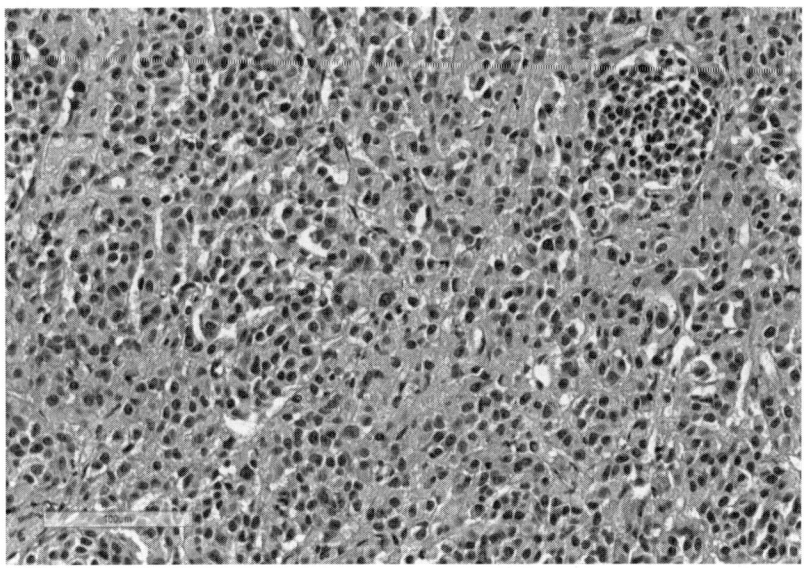

Figure 9. Malignant melanomas show proliferation of atypical, pleomorphic epithelioid cells. In the absence of melanin pigment and junctional/epidermal component, this tumor overlaps morphologically with epithlioid MPNSTs (hematoxylin and eosin, original magnification 200X).

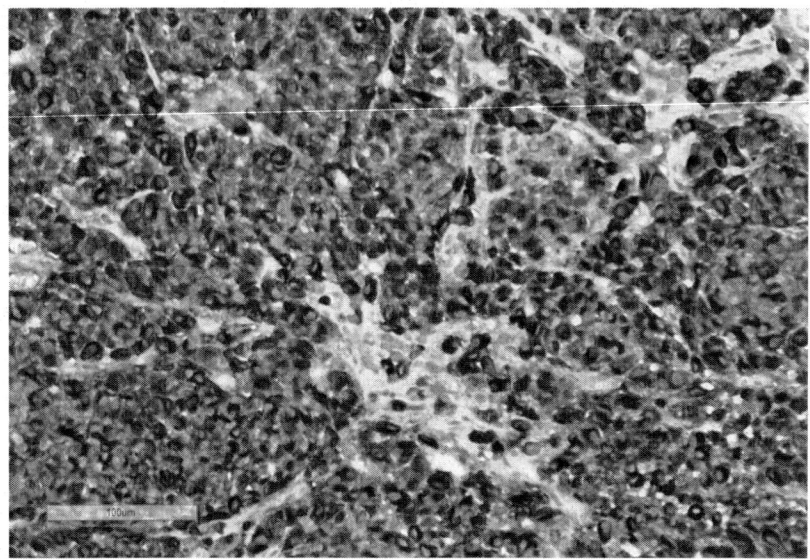

Figure 10. Same case in figure 9 showing diffuse cytoplasmic staining with melan A, a melanocytic marker. This marker should be negative in all cases of epithelioid MPNSTS (original magnification 200X).

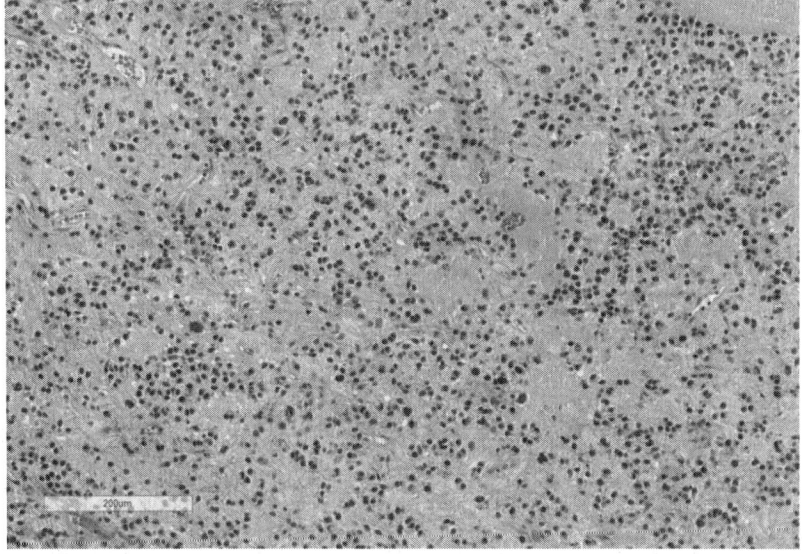

Figure 11. Myoepithelial carcinomas, similar to epithlioid MPNSTs, show proliferation of epithelioid cells with atypia. The stroma can be predominantly myxoid, which can add to the challenge in distinguishing them from epithlioid MPNSTs (hematoxylin and eosin, original magnification 100X).

Myoepithelial carcinomas should be considered in the differential diagnosis too, as they can marked by a proliferation of atypical epithelioid cells with vesicular nuclei and prominent nucleoli, similar to eMPNSTs [31]. They also commonly have a myxoid stroma and the majority of them show S-100 expression (Figure 11) [3, 31]. Up to 20% of the cases can show loss of SMARCB1 expression by immunohistochemistry [23]. Nevertheless, their reactivity to various epithelial markers (cytokeratin and/or EMA) and myogenic markers (calponin and SMA) help differentiate them from eMPNSTs (Figure 12) [3, 31]. Fluorescence In situ hybridization (FISH) for *EWSR1* gene rearrangement can be useful in confirming some of the cases, as it is detected in around 50% of myoepithelial carcinomas [31]. Epithelioid sarcomas, proximal – type, are characterized by a large, atypical epithelioid cells (Figure 13) [23]. They occur most frequently around the pelvic girdle in young adults [23]. The majority of epithelioid sarcomas show loss of SMARCB1 expression [23]; nevertheless, the rest of the immunohistochemical expression profile is fairly different than eMPNSTs, as they are usually S-100 negative and cytokeratin/EMA positive (Figure 14) [3, 23].

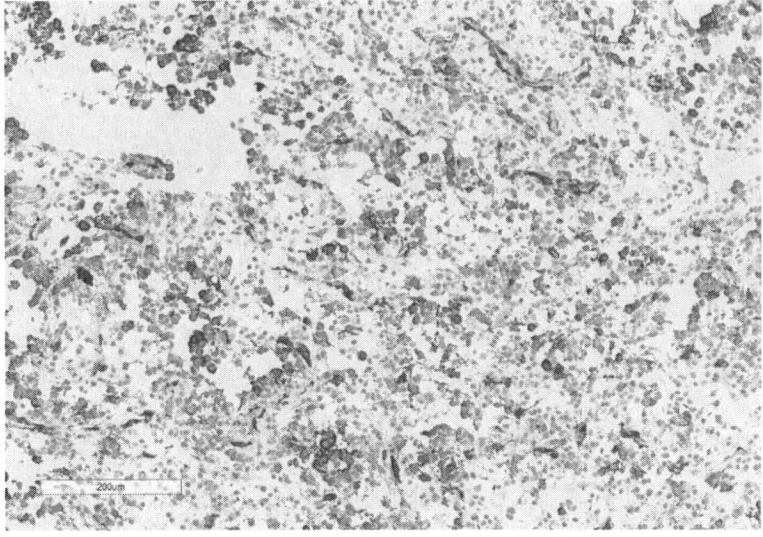

Figure 12. The majority of myoepithelial carcinomas show strong cytoplasmic positivity with smooth muscle actin (SMA) (original magnification 100X).

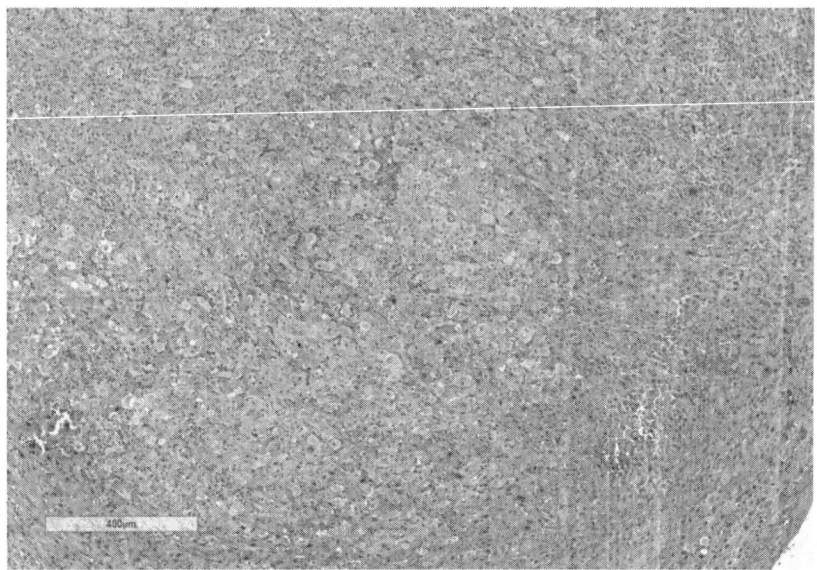

Figure 13. Epithelioid sarcoma, proximal type, demonstrate proliferation of large cells with atypical nuclei and moderate amount of eosinophilic cytoplasm (hematoxylin and eosin, original magnification 50X).

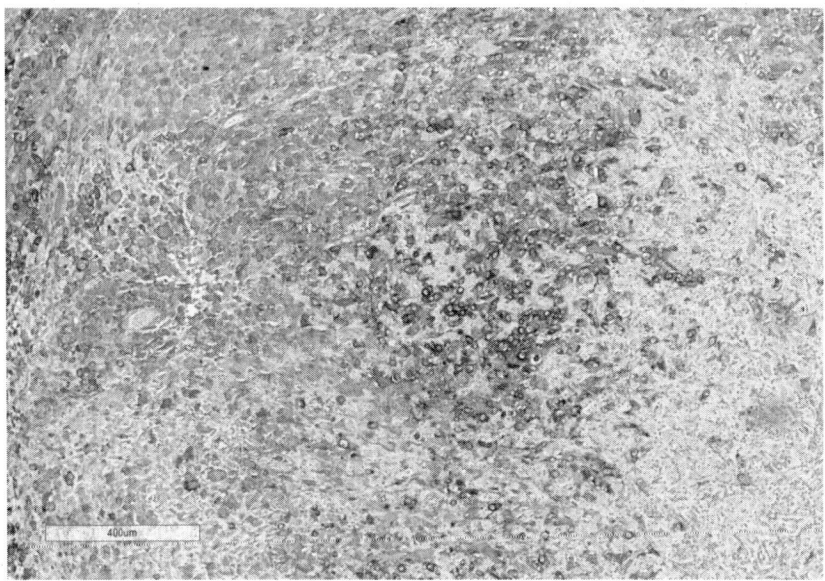

Figure 14. The case in figure 13 of epithelioid sarcoma shows cytoplasmic positive with cytokeratins AE1/AE3, a feature that distinguish them from epithelioid MPNSTs (original magnification 50X).

Metastatic poorly differentiated carcinoma is another consideration, but this can be easily distinguished by the common association with prior history of carcinoma, and distinctive immunohistochemical profile including expression of cytokeratins/EMA, absence of S-100 expression, and the frequent expression of other primary site specific markers [3].

Prognosis and Treatment

Data about the prognosis of eMPNSTs is still limited due to their rarity; nevertheless, multiple case reports and case series report aggressive behavior with local recurrence and metastasis [12]. The data on the extent of this aggressive behavior is conflicting. Older reports show a behavior similar to conventional MPNSTs with high risk of local recurrence and distant metastasis (up to around 50% of the cases in some series) [12]; this finding is contradicted in more recent and larger case series studies [3, 5, 6]. Older reports also showed that superficial tumors have a decreased risk of metastasis and a better prognosis than deep-seated tumors [4], a finding also described in conventional MPNSTs [32]. A more recent, larger series by Jo et al. failed to reproduce this difference [3]. One possible explanation can be that deep-seated tumors are more easily resected with wide margins nowadays than before. Some authors also raise the possibility that some of the superficial tumors are in fact epithelioid schwannomas, provided that this entity was not characterized until more recently [3], which can also explain some of the differences about the extent of the aggressive behavior of eMPNSTs between older and newer reports. The current proposed sarcoma histologic grading criteria do not correlate well with the behavior of either eMPNSTs or conventional MPNSTs [16]. As was mentioned in previous sections, eMPNSTs are rarely associated with NF1, and whether cases associated with NF1 have a worse behavior or not is controversial, given the varied data in the literature [33-35].

Similar to most soft tissue sarcomas, the standard of therapy for MPNSTs, including eMPNSTs, is surgical resection of the tumor with wide negative margins. Positive margins are a significant predictor of local recurrence [36]. Radiation, though its role is still not well defined, can be considered preoperatively (neoadjuvant) for bigger lesions (>5cm) or adjuvant for cases with positive margins [36]. Adjuvant chemotherapy is commonly used, with a fair response at best [36]. The observation that epidermal growth factor receptor (EGFR) amplification was found in a subset of MPNSTs led to many clinical trials looking into EGFR inhibitors as a potential treatment modality [36]. Although all clinical trials to date failed to show response [36], these efforts are leading the way to explore better-targeted agents against this aggressive disease. Such data about eMPNSTs, in particular, are lacking due to the few numbers of cases, with the largest series to date being comprised of only 63 cases [3]. eMPNSTs tend to have a more superficial location and smaller size compared to conventional MPNSTs [3-6], which makes complete surgical excision even more at the forefront of curing this disease.

REFERENCES

[1] McCormack, L. J., Hazard, J. B., Dlckson, J. A. Malignant epithelioid neurilemoma (schwannoma). *Cancer*, 1954; 7(4):725 - 728.

[2] Ducatman, B. S., Scheithauer, B. W., Piepgras, D. G., Reiman, H. M., Ilstrup, D. M. Malignant peripheral nerve sheath tumors. A clinicopathologic study of 120 cases. *Cancer*, 1986; 57(10):2006 - 2021.

[3] Jo, V. Y., Fletcher, C. D. M. Epithelioid malignant peripheral nerve sheath tumor: Clinicopathologic analysis of 63 cases. *Am. J. Surg. Pathol.*, 2015; 39(5):673 - 682.

[4] Laskin, W. B., Weiss, S. W., Bratthauer, G. L. Epithelioid variant of malignant peripheral nerve sheath tumor (malignant epithelioid schwannoma). *Am. J. Surg. Pathol.*, 1991; 15(12):1136 - 1145.

[5] Rekhi, B., Kosemehmetoglu, K., Tezel, G. G., Dervisoglu, S. Clinicopathologic features and immunohistochemical spectrum of 11 cases of epithelioid malignant peripheral nerve sheath tumors,

including INI1/SMARCB1 results and BRAF V600E analysis. *APMIS*, 2017; 125(8):679 - 689.

[6] Luzar, B., Shanesmith, R., Ramakrishnan, R., Fisher, C., Calonje, E. Cutaneous epithelioid malignant peripheral nerve sheath tumour: A clinicopathological analysis of 11 cases. *Histopathology*, 2016; 68(2):286 - 296.

[7] Agaimy, A., Stachel, K. D., Jüngert, J. et al. Malignant epithelioid peripheral nerve sheath tumor with prominent reticular/microcystic pattern in a child: A low-grade neoplasm with 18-years follow-up. *Appl. Immunohistochem. Mol. Morphol.*, 2014; 22(8):627 - 633.

[8] Wu, L., Deng, X., Yang, C., Xu, Y. Spinal intradural malignant peripheral nerve sheath tumor in a child with neurofibromatosis type 2: The first reported case and literature review. *Turk. Neurosurg.*, 2014; 24(1):135 - 139.

[9] Patra, S., Ayyanar, P., Padhi, S., Purkait, S., Muduly, D. K., Samal, S. C. Epithelioid malignant peripheral nerve sheath tumor (epithelioid-MPNST) presenting as bleeding rectal polyp: A case report with systematic literature review. *Am. J. Case Rep.*, 2019; 20:1175 - 1181.

[10] Hirokawa, M., Shimizu, M., Fukuoka, K. et al. Intraosseous epithelioid malignant peripheral nerve sheath tumor of the phalanx. Case report. *APMIS*, 1999; 107(4):401 - 403.

[11] Chee, D. W. Y., Peh, W. C. G., Shek, T. W. H. Pictorial essay: Imaging of peripheral nerve sheath tumours. *Can. Assoc. Radiol. J.*, 2011; 62(3):176 - 182.

[12] Lodding, P., Kindblom, L. G., Angervall, L. Epithelioid malignant schwannoma. A study of 14 cases. *Virchows Arch. A Pathol. Anat. Histopathol.*, 1986; 409(4):433 - 451.

[13] Cheng, J. X., Tretiakova, M., Gong, C., Mandal, S., Krausz, T., Taxy, J. B. Renal medullary carcinoma: Rhabdoid features and the absence of INI1 expression as markers of aggressive behavior. *Mod. Pathol.*, 2008.

[14] Laskin, W. B., Fetsch, J. F., Lasota, J., Miettinen, M. Benign epithelioid peripheral nerve sheath tumors of the soft tissues:

Clinicopathologic spectrum of 33 cases. *Am. J. Surg. Pathol.*, 2005; 29(1):39 - 51.
[15] Hart, J., Gardner, J. M., Edgar, M., Weiss, S. W. Epithelioid schwannomas: An analysis of 58 cases including atypical variants. *Am. J. Surg. Pathol.*, 2016; 40(5):704 - 713.
[16] Coindre, J. M., Terrier, P., Guillou, L. et al. Predictive value of grade for metastasis development in the main histologic types of adult soft tissue sarcomas: A study of 1240 patients from the French Federation of Cancer Centers sarcoma group. *Cancer*, 2001; 91(10):1914 - 1926.
[17] Kolberg, M., Høland, M., Agesen, T. H. et al. Survival meta-analyses for >1800 malignant peripheral nerve sheath tumor patients with and without neurofibromatosis type 1. *Neuro Oncol.*, 2013; 15(2):135 - 147.
[18] Thway, K., Fisher, C. Malignant peripheral nerve sheath tumor: Pathology and genetics. *Ann. Diagn. Pathol.*, 2014; 18(2):109 - 116.
[19] Schaefer, I. M., Fletcher, C. D. M., Hornick, J. L. Loss of H3K27 trimethylation distinguishes malignant peripheral nerve sheath tumors from histologic mimics. *Mod. Pathol.*, 2016; 29(1):4 - 13.
[20] Prieto-Granada, C. N., Wiesner, T., Messina, J. L., Jungbluth, A. A., Chi, P., Antonescu, C. R. Loss of H3K27me3 expression is a highly sensitive marker for sporadic and radiation-induced MPNST. *Am. J. Surg. Pathol.*, 2016; 40(4):479 - 489.
[21] Schaefer, I. M., Dong, F., Garcia, E. P., Fletcher, C. D. M., Jo, V. Y. Recurrent SMARCB1 inactivation in epithelioid malignant peripheral nerve sheath tumors. *Am. J. Surg. Pathol.*, 2019; 43(6):835 - 843.
[22] Sápi, Z., Papp, G., Szendrői, M. et al. Epigenetic regulation of SMARCB1 By miR-206, -381 and -671-5p is evident in a variety of SMARCB1 immunonegative soft tissue sarcomas, while miR-765 appears specific for epithelioid sarcoma. A miRNA study of 223 soft tissue sarcomas. *Genes, Chromosom Cancer*, 2016; 55(10):786 - 802.
[23] Hornick, J. L., Dal Cin, P., Fletcher, C. D. M. Loss of INI1 expression is characteristic of both conventional and proximal-type epithelioid sarcoma. *Am. J. Surg. Pathol.*, 2009; 33(4):542 - 550.

[24] Jo, V. Y., Fletcher, C. D. M. SMARCB1/INI1 loss in epithelioid schwannoma. *Am. J. Surg. Pathol.*, 2017; 41(8):1013 - 1022.
[25] Haberler, C., Laggner, U., Slavc, I. et al. Immunohistochemical analysis of INI1 protein in malignant pediatric CNS tumors: Lack of INI1 in atypical teratoid/rhabdoid tumors and in a fraction of primitive neuroectodermal tumors without rhabdoid phenotype. *Am. J. Surg. Pathol.*, 2006; 30(11):1462 - 1468.
[26] Lee, W., Teckie, S., Wiesner, T. et al. PRC2 is recurrently inactivated through EED or SUZ12 loss in malignant peripheral nerve sheath tumors. *Nat. Genet.*, 2014; 46(11):1227 - 1232.
[27] De Raedt, T., Beert, E., Pasmant, E. et al. PRC2 loss amplifies Ras-driven transcription and confers sensitivity to BRD4-based therapies. *Nature*, 2014; 514(7521):247 - 251.
[28] Martinez, A. P., Fritchie, K. J. Update on peripheral nerve sheath tumors. *Surg. Pathol. Clin.*, 2019; 12(1):1 - 19.
[29] Blessing, K., Sanders, D. S. A., Grant, J. J. H. Comparison of immunohistochemical staining of the novel antibody melan- A with S100 protein and HMB-45 in malignant melanoma and melanoma variants. *Histopathology*, 1998; 32(2):139 - 146.
[30] Wick, M. R., Gru, A. A. Metastatic melanoma: Pathologic characterization, current treatment, and complications of therapy. *Semin. Diagn. Pathol.*, 2016; 33(4):204 - 218.
[31] Jo, V. Y., Fletcher, C. D. M. Myoepithelial neoplasms of soft tissue: an updated review of the clinicopathologic, immunophenotypic, and genetic features. *Head Neck Pathol.*, 2015; 9(1):32 - 38.
[32] Valentin, T., Le Cesne, A., Ray-Coquard, I. et al. Management and prognosis of malignant peripheral nerve sheath tumors: The experience of the French Sarcoma Group (GSF-GETO). *Eur. J. Cancer*, 2016; 56(2016):77 - 84.
[33] Yuan, Z., Xu, L., Zhao, Z. et al. Clinicopathological features and prognosis of malignant peripheral nerve sheath tumor: A retrospective study of 159 cases from 1999 to 2016. *Oncotarget*, 2017; 8(62):104785 - 104795.

[34] Hagel, C., Zils, U., Peiper, M. et al. Histopathology and clinical outcome of NF1-associated vs. sporadic malignant peripheral nerve sheath tumors. *J. Neurooncol.*, 2007; 82(2):187 - 192.

[35] Porter, D. E., Prasad, V., Foster, L., Dall, G. F., Birch, R., Grimer, R. J. Survival in malignant peripheral nerve sheath tumours: A comparison between sporadic and neurofibromatosis type 1-associated tumours. *Sarcoma*, 2009; 2009.

[36] Kim, A. R., Stewart, D. R., Reilly, K. M., Viskochil, D., Miettinen, M. M., Wideman, B. C. Malignant peripheral nerve sheath tumors state of the science: Leveraging clinical and biological insights into effective therapies. *Sarcoma*, 2017; 2017(Table 1).

In: Nerve Sheath Tumors
Editor: Richard A. Prayson

ISBN: 978-1-53617-366-6
© 2020 Nova Science Publishers, Inc.

Chapter 2

COLONIC PERINEURIOMA: A REVIEW OF CLINICOPATHOLOGIC FEATURES

Lanisha D. Fuller, MD and Richard A. Prayson[*], MD, MEd

Department of Anatomic Pathology, Cleveland Clinic, Cleveland, OH, US

ABSTRACT

Perineuriomas are benign neoplasms of the peripheral nerve sheath that are comprised entirely of perineurial cells. These tumors may arise within the intraneural compartment, formerly known as localized hypertrophic neuropathy, or in the soft tissue compartment, formerly known as storiform perineural fibroma. Soft tissue perineuriomas are usually found in the subcutis of extremities and the trunk. Infrequently however, they occur in the gastrointestinal tract, especially in the distal colon. Colonic perineuriomas typically present as small mucosal polyps and are discovered incidentally during screening colonoscopy. Histologically, they are marked by a proliferation of elongated perineurial cells growing in fascicles or bundles that separate the crypts. Perineurial

---

[*] Corresponding Author's Email: praysor@ccf.org; Fax: 216-445-6967.

cells are epithelial membrane antigen (EMA), claudin-1 and glucose transporter-1 (GLUT1) positive while negative for S-100 protein, which allows their distinction from other peripheral nerve sheath tumors. They are negative for muscle markers and c-KIT which allows distinction from more common spindle cell neoplasms encountered in the gastrointestinal tract. Differential diagnostic considerations include other nerve sheath tumors as well as leiomyoma and gastrointestinal stromal tumor (GIST).

INTRODUCTION

Perineuriomas are benign neoplasms of the peripheral nerve sheath. What sets them apart from other peripheral nerve sheath tumors is that they are composed entirely of neoplastic perineurial cells. Depending on whether a perineurioma occurs in a nerve or outside of a nerve in the soft tissue, it is classified as either an intraneural or soft tissue perineurioma. Soft tissue perineuriomas were formerly known as "storiform perineurial fibroma". Intraneural perineuriomas were thought to be a reactive process and were formerly known as "reactive hypertrophic neuropathy". However, abnormalities of chromosome 22 have been shown in intraneural as well as soft tissue perineuriomas [1], supporting a neoplastic nature. While intraneural perineuriomas usually involve peripheral nerves of younger patients [2], soft tissue perineuriomas commonly occur in the subcutis of the lower extremities and trunk in middle-aged and older individuals [1]. Soft tissue perineuriomas infrequently involve visceral organs. Of all visceral organs, they are most commonly encountered in the gastrointestinal tract [1]. Most perineuriomas of the gastrointestinal tract are found in the distal colon [3, 4], which however might be a bias due to established screening procedures of the colon and rectum.

Perineuriomas were first described in 1978 by Lazarus and Trombetta, when they examined the ultrastructure of a tumor that previously had been classified as neurofibroma by light microscopy [5]. They described a tumor composed of spindle cells with thin cytoplasmic processes and numerous surface vesicles surrounded by a collagen rich matrix. The cells had either no basement membrane or simply a fragmented one. They found that these characteristics were similar to those found in perineurial cells of small peripheral nerves in the skin and suggested perineurioma as a new entity.

CLINICAL ASPECTS AND OUTCOME

Colonic perineuriomas are usually asymptomatic and incidentally diagnosed during screening colonoscopy or workup of other bowel conditions. About 69% of cases were found during routine colonoscopy, 4% during screening colonoscopy for patients with previous rectal cancers, 13% for gastrointestinal bleeding, 9% for abdominal pain and the remainder of cases during workup of other conditions [6]. In a study, two institutions found that about 0.2% of the colonic polyps they examine yearly are colonic perineuriomas [7]. About three quarters present as small sessile mucosal polyps distal to the splenic flexure [6, 8]. The mean age at diagnosis is 60 years (range 35 - 87 years) with a slight female predominance (F:M = 1.3) [6]. They are usually sporadic lesions and not associated with any hereditary tumor syndromes [9]. Only few cases have been reported of perineuriomas in neurofibromatosis type 1 patients [10] which most likely were coincidental. However, so far no cases of colonic perineurioma in conjunction with hereditary tumor syndromes have been reported. They are benign and do not recur after gross total excision [11]. So far, no cases of metastasis or malignant progression have been reported [6]. There is no need for follow-up after complete resection.

WHAT THE LITERATURE SAYS
ABOUT COLONIC PERINEURIOMAS

In 2004, Eslami-Varzaneh et al. described 14 cases of a distinctive type of mucosal polyp in the colon which was composed of monomorphic spindle cells in the lamina propria that separated and disorganized the colonic crypts but showed no necrosis or significant mitotic activity [7]. All lesions were solitary and not associated with a known polyposis syndrome. Ten of the cases were associated with adenomata and/or hyperplastic polyps at different sites. Three cases showed close association with hyperplastic polyps. Immunohistochemical stains were strongly positive for vimentin and focally weakly positive for CD34 in a subset of cases; all cases were negative for epithelial membrane antigen (EMA), smooth muscle actin, desmin, CD31, Bcl-2, c-KIT and S-100 protein. Electron microscopy was performed on two of the cases and revealed spindled cells surrounded by collagen fibers with sparse cytoplasmic organelles and many intermediate filaments. The cells lacked a basal lamina, dense bodies, and pinocytic vesicles. In light of their findings, they hypothesized that the cells showed fibroblastic differentiation and designated them as "fibroblastic polyps". They deduced that the absence of EMA staining excluded perineurioma from the differentials.

In 2005, Hornick and Fletcher were the first to describe perineuriomas in the gastrointestinal tract [4]. The study included ten perineuriomas arising in the intestine, eight of which were mucosal polyps arising in the colon. They described them as lesions composed of bland spindle cells with ovoid to tapered nuclei and pale cytoplasm that entrapped colonic crypts. The background was composed of fine collagenous stroma. No cytologic atypia, pleomorphism or mitotic activity was seen. Immunohistochemistry performed on the ten cases showed positivity for EMA in nine, claudin-1 in four, and CD34 in two of the cases; all were negative for S-100 protein, glial fibrillary acidic protein (GFAP), neurofilament protein, smooth muscle actin (SMA), desmin, caldesmon, c-KIT, and pan-keratin. They then examined the EMA negative tumor electron microscopically which revealed spindle cells with long bipolar cytoplasmic processes and abundant pinocytotic vesicles, surrounded by a discontinuous basal lamina. These findings correlated with previous descriptions of perineurioma. Hornick and Fletcher also saw similarities in cytomorphology of colonic perineuriomas and previously described fibroblastic polyps and noted frequent entrapment of crypts in both lesions.

A subsequent study by Groisman and Polak-Charcon in 2008 found that some colonic perineuriomas have limited or weak expression of EMA [8]. They performed immunohistochemical staining for EMA, claudin-1,

GLUT-1 and collagen type IV on 28 cases with histologic features of fibroblastic polyps/perineuriomas of the colon and rectum. All lesions were composed of fascicles or bundles of bland spindle cells with plump or slender nuclei and pale indistinct cytoplasm that separated the crypts. Immunohistochemistry revealed positivity for EMA in 26 of the lesions. The staining was focal and weak with a membranous pattern, even though extended heat-induced antigen retrieval was performed before staining and a detection amplification kit was used. However, with these methods, eight cases that previously did not stain using standard staining protocol, were now positive. Claudin-1, too, was positive in 26 cases and GLUT-1 was positive in all cases. In contrast to EMA, claudin-1 and GLUT 1 stained strongly and diffusely with a membranous, granular pattern despite only using a standard staining protocol. All cases also showed strong, membranous and granular staining for collagen type IV. Electron microscopy of four cases, including two cases that were previously classified as fibroblastic polyps, revealed abundant collagen fibers in every case. The tumor cells showed features of perineurial differentiation, characterized by long and thin cytoplasmic processes, a discontinuous basal lamina, and pinocytotic vesicles. They concluded that extended antigen retrieval methods, signal amplification and/or the use of at least two perineurial markers should be implemented to reach an accurate diagnosis and hypothesized that some, if not all, lesions previously classified as fibroblastic polyps of the colon could in fact be perineuriomas. This hypothesis is supported by findings like those of Zamecnik and Chlumska, who stained five cases previously classified as fibroblastic polyps with claudin-1 and GLUT-1 [12]. Additionally, they repeated staining for EMA with a higher antibody concentration and found that three cases were positive for EMA, four for claudin-1 and all cases for GLUT-1. Every case was positive for at least two of the markers. They then examined the lesion that was positive for all three markers electron microscopically which revealed findings similar to those of Groisman and Polak-Charcon and typical of perineurial cell differentiation [8]. They also stated that, despite specimen preservation having been suboptimal for electron microscopy, they were able to find areas of unquestionable basal lamina on cell processes and some pinocytotic vesicles and primitive cell junctions.

GROSS AND MICROSCOPIC PATHOLOGY

Grossly, colonic mucosal perineuriomas form well-circumscribed, small, sessile polyps up to 1.5 cm in size with a smooth surface [4, 13, 14]. Even though most are sessile lesions, pedunculated polyps have also been reported [6, 8], indicating a variety in gross appearance. So far only solitary colonic perineuriomas have been reported [6, 7].

Histologically, they present as a well-circumscribed, unencapsulated, proliferation of uniform, plump cells with pale eosinophilic cytoplasm and indistinct cell borders, embedded within a delicate collagenous stroma in the lamina propria mucosae (Figure 1) [3, 4, 6-8]. Akin to soft tissue perineuriomas at other locations, they show a variety of growth patterns, including, fascicular, bundled and storiform. Often, they also show a whorling growth pattern around crypts [9]. The nuclei are oval to spindled with inconspicuous nucleoli. No nuclear atypia, necrosis or significant mitotic activity are seen (Figure 2).

The cells expand the lamina propria, separating and entrapping the crypts. Most cases have a rim of uninvolved lamina propria between the spindle cells and the surface epithelium [3].

ANCILLARY STUDIES

Because of their histomorphologic similarity to other nerve sheath tumors and spindle cell lesions, immunohistochemical stains can be useful tools in helping to differentiate between them. Just like perineuriomas at other locations, they show diffuse and strong immunoreactivity for glucose transporter-1 (GLUT1) and claudin-1.

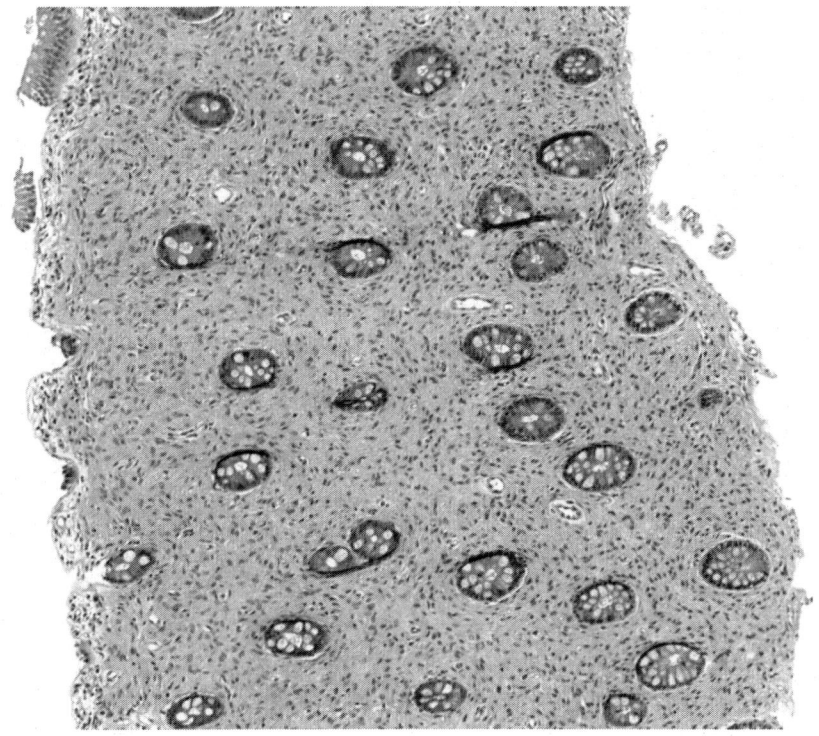

Figure 1. Colonic perineurioma. A proliferation of plump, oval cells expands the lamina propria mucosae and separates the colonic crypts (hematoxylin and eosin, original magnification 100X).

Perineuriomas are embedded in a delicate collagenous stroma that is composed of type IV collagen, as can be demonstrated by antibodies against the same. Ki-67 staining shows low proliferation rates, usually staining less than 1% of nuclei [6]. Usually, they are nonreactive for markers against smooth muscle actin (SMA), S-100 protein, CD34, desmin, and c-KIT (CD117). However, weak, focal positivity for CD34 has been reported [7, 15]. Their nonreactivity toward S-100 protein is especially helpful in distinguishing perineuriomas from other nerve sheath tumors. The classic positive marker for intraneural, as well as soft tissue perineuriomas is epithelial membrane antigen (EMA) (Figure 3). While colonic perineuriomas stain with EMA, they sometimes only show focal weak, membranous reactivity to it, making it difficult to discern on low power.

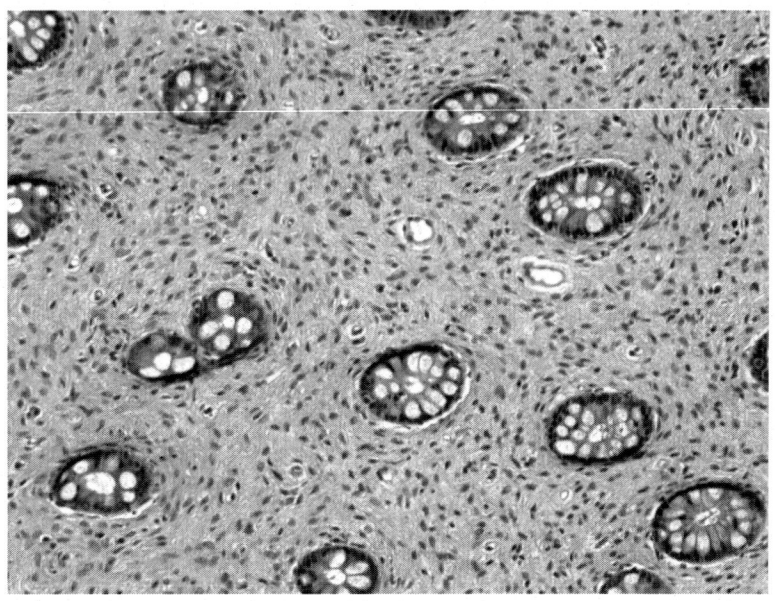

Figure 2. Colonic perineurioma. Higher power view demonstrates the bland spindle cells without nuclear atypia. Note the fine collagenous meshwork the cells are embedded in (hematoxylin and eosin, original magnification 200X).

This might be a problem, when one relies solely on EMA to exclude perineurioma. Because of the weak and limited EMA expression, more extensive antigen retrieval methods and signal amplification might help in detecting staining. Authors have also suggested using more than one marker of perineurial differentiation to reach an accurate diagnosis [8].

Electron microscopic findings are the same as those of soft tissue perineuriomas at other locations. Embedded in a collagenous stroma and surrounded by a wispy, discontinuous basal lamina are spindle cells with long, thin cytoplasmic processes, pinocytotic vesicles and few organelles [4, 8].

COLONIC PERINEURIOMAS AND SERRATED POLYPS

About 75% of colonic perineuriomas are associated with serrated or hyperplastic changes of the mucosal epithelium [6].

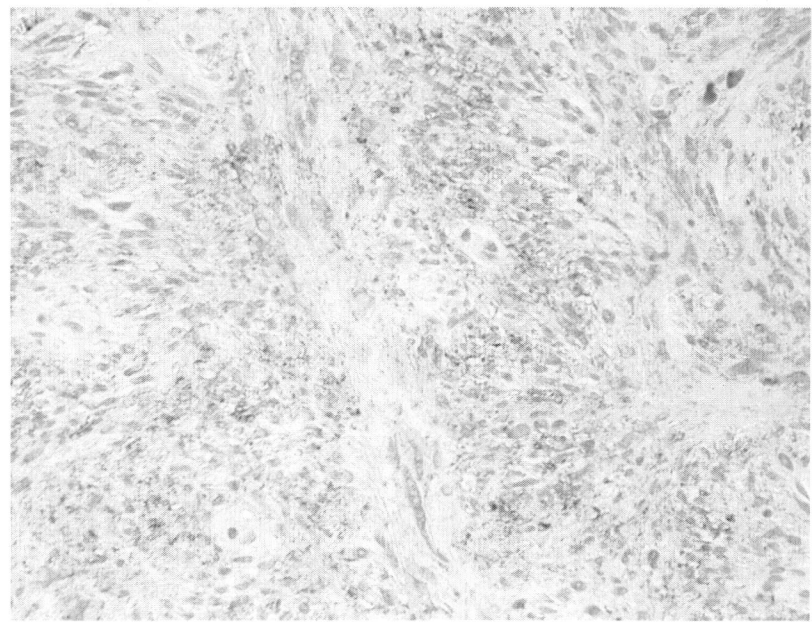

Figure 3. Colonic perineurioma. The cells show diffuse positivity for EMA (EMA, original magnification 400X).

Likewise, a study found that 6.5% of sessile serrated adenomas were associated with at least focal perineurial proliferations [16]. The epithelial changes in most cases resembled those of a microvesicular hyperplastic polyp [6]. Molecular analysis for BRAF V600E mutations detected mutations in about 60% of cases with combined perineuroma and serrated epithelium [17]. A small subset of lesions showed BRAF mutations other than V600E. In contrast, mutational analysis of perineuriomas without epithelial serration detected no BRAF mutations. Immunoreactivity to a BRAF V600E mutation-specific antibody in the serrated epithelium but not in the perineurial proliferation or nonserrated crypt epithelium has been demonstrated [6]. Also, separation into epithelial and perineurial components via microdissection has shown BRAF mutations in the serrated epithelium, but not in the perineurial proliferation [18]. A question that remains is whether the perineurial proliferation in the combined cases is neoplastic or represents a reactive process. Mutational analysis including abnormalities of chromosome 22 have not been performed on the perineurial proliferations in these combined lesions.

DIFFERENTIAL DIAGNOSTIC CONSIDERATIONS

The list of spindle cell lesions to consider as differentials for perineurioma is long and distinguishing between the entities without immunohistochemical staining can be challenging. In the gastrointestinal tract, differentials can be narrowed down according to which lesions are more commonly encountered, and include but are not limited to gastrointestinal stromal tumor (GIST), leiomyoma, schwannoma, neurofibroma and ganglioneuroma.

Even though uncommon in the colon, a differential diagnostic consideration should include GIST, since it has the potential to be malignant. The spindle cell variant of GIST can morphologically look similar to perineurioma. They present as masses formed by fascicles of plump spindle cells with eosinophilic cytoplasm. Unlike leiomyoma and perineurioma, they are usually centered within the muscularis propria. Immunohistochemical stains for DOG1 and c-KIT are usually positive.

A more common type of mesenchymal tumor in the colon is leiomyoma [19]. It is a benign smooth muscle tumor that arises from the muscularis mucosa. Histologically, it forms sharply demarcated nodules of mature, disorganized smooth muscle bundles that do not entrap crypts [13]. In contrast to perineurioma, the cytoplasm is usually brightly eosinophilic. Strong and diffuse positivity for SMA and desmin is characteristic.

Ganglioneuroma is a benign peripheral nerve sheath tumor that histologically has ill-defined margins and can entrap crypts [4, 13]. It is composed of spindled Schwannian cells and a variable numbers of either nested or individually admixed mature ganglion cells. No significant atypia, mitoses, or necrosis should be present in either component. Staining for S-100 protein should stain the Schwann as well as ganglion cells.

Colonic schwannoma is a nonencapsulated proliferation of neoplastic Schwann cells with spindled nuclei that characteristically is surrounded by a lymphoid cuff. Unlike their extraintestinal counterparts, they often lack typical Antoni A and B zonation and Verocay bodies. Similar to GIST, it arises within the muscularis propria. The cells are diffusely and strongly positive for S-100 protein.

While gastrointestinal neurofibromas are rare in the general population, they occur more frequently in patients with neurofibromatosis type 1 [6, 9]. They can affect any layer of the bowel wall and consist of S-100 protein positive Schwann cells with wavy nuclei, fibroblasts and perineurial cells.

REFERENCES

[1] Perry, Arie and Daniel J. Brat. 2010. "Perineurioma". In *Practical Surgical Neuropathology*: A Volume in the Pattern Recognition Series. London: Elsevier Health Sciences. (Scheithauer, Woodruff and Spinner, 2010, 260 - 67).

[2] Alkhaili, Jaber, Adeline Cambon-Binder and Zoubir Belkheyar. 2018. "Intraneural Perineurioma – a Retrospective Study of 19 Patients". *Pan African Medical Journal,* 30:275.

[3] Groisman, Gabriel M., Dov Hershkovitz, Michael Vieth and Edmond Sabo. 2013. "Colonic Perineuriomas With and Without Crypt Serration". *The American Journal of Surgical Pathology,* 37, no. 5: 745 - 51.

[4] Hornick, Jason L. and Christopher D. M. Fletcher. 2005. "Intestinal Perineuriomas". *The American Journal of Surgical Pathology*, 29, no. 7: 859 - 65.

[5] Lazarus, Sydney S. and Louis D. Trombetta. 1978. "Ultrastructural Identification of a Benign Perineurial Cell Tumor". *Cancer,* 41, no. 5: 1823 - 29.

[6] Wyk, Abraham Christoffel Van, Hennie Van Zyl and Jonathan Rigby. 2018. "Colonic Perineurioma (Benign Fibroblastic Polyp): Case Report and Review of the Literature". *Diagnostic Pathology,* 13, no. 1: 16.

[7] Eslami-Varzaneh, Fatima, Kay Washington, Marie E. Robert, Michael Kashgarian, John R. Goldblum and Dhanpat Jain. 2004. "Benign Fibroblastic Polyps of the Colon". *The American Journal of Surgical Pathology*, 28, no. 3: 374 - 78.

[8] Groisman, Gabriel M. and Sylvie Polak-Charcon. 2008. "Fibroblastic Polyp of the Colon and Colonic Perineurioma: 2 Names for a Single Entity?" *The American Journal of Surgical Pathology*, 32, no. 7: 1088 - 94.

[9] Mccarthy, Aoife J., Dipti M. Karamchandani and Runjan Chetty. 2018. "Neural and Neurogenic Tumours of the Gastroenteropancreaticobiliary Tract". *Journal of Clinical Pathology*, 71, no. 7: 565 - 78.

[10] Schaefer, Inga-Marie, Philipp Ströbel, Aung Thiha, Jan Martin Sohns, Christian Mühlfeld, Stefan Küffer, Gunther Felmerer, Adam Stepniewski, Silke Pauli and Abbas Agaimy. 2013. "Soft tissue perineurioma and other unusual tumors in a patient with neurofibromatosis type 1". *International Journal of Clinical and Experimental Pathology*, 6, no 12: 3003 - 3008.

[11] Groisman, Gabriel, Mary Amar and Meir Alona. 2009, "Early Colonic Perineurioma: A Report of 11 Cases". *International Journal of Surgical Pathology*, 18, no. 4: 292 - 97.

[12] Zamecnik, Michal and Alena Chlumska. 2006. "Perineurioma Versus Fibroblastic Polyp of the Colon". *The American Journal of Surgical Pathology*, 30, no. 10: 1337 - 39.

[13] Otani, Tomoyuki, Kinta Hatakeyama, Emi Ohtani, Susumu Nakayama, Takashi Fujimoto and Chiho Ohbayashi. 2018. "A Colonic Perineurioma". Clinical Medicine Insights. *Pathology*, 11: 117955571881591. Accessed October 24, 2019. doi: 10.1177/1179555718815918.

[14] Jama, Guled M., Matthew Evans, Muhammad W. Fazal and Deepak Singh-Ranger. 2018. "Perineurioma of the Sigmoid Colon". *BMJ Case Reports*, 2018:bcr-2018-227170. Accessed October 24, 2019. doi: 10.1136/bcr-2018-227170.

[15] Fujino, Yasuteru, Naoki Muguruma, Shinji Kitamura, Yasuhiro Mitsui, Tetsuo Kimura, Hiroshi Miyamoto, Hisanori Uehara, Koichi Kataoka and Tetsuji Takayama. 2014. "Perineurioma in the Sigmoid Colon Diagnosed and Treated by Endoscopic Resection". *Clinical Journal of Gastroenterology,* 7, no. 5: 392 - 96.

[16] Pai, Reetesh K., Amirkaveh Mojtahed, Robert V. Rouse, Roy M. Soetikno, Tonya Kaltenbach, Lisa Ma, Daniel A. Arber, Thomas P. Plesec, John R. Goldblum and Rish K. Pai. 2011. "Histologic and Molecular Analyses of Colonic Perineurial-like Proliferations in Serrated Polyps". *The American Journal of Surgical Pathology,* 35, no. 9: 1373 - 80.

[17] Agaimy, Abbas, Robert Stoehr, Michael Vieth and Arndt Hartmann. 2010. "Benign Serrated Colorectal Fibroblastic Polyps/Intramucosal Perineuriomas Are True Mixed Epithelial-Stromal Polyps (Hybrid Hyperplastic Polyp/Mucosal Perineurioma) With Frequent BRAF Mutations". *The American Journal of Surgical Pathology,* 34, no. 11: 1663 - 71.

[18] Erlenbach-Wünsch, Katharina, Michel Bihl, Arndt Hartmann, Gabriel M. Groisman, Michael Vieth and Abbas Agaimy. 2018. "Serrated Epithelial Colorectal Polyps (Hyperplastic Polyps, Sessile Serrated Adenomas) with Perineurial Stroma: Clinicopathological and Molecular Analysis of a New Series". *Annals of Diagnostic Pathology,* 35: 48 - 52.

[19] Odze, Robert D. and John R. Goldblum. 2009. *Surgical Pathology of the GI Tract, Liver, Biliary Tract and Pancreas: Expert Consult: Online and Print.* London: Elsevier Health Sciences. (Hornick and Odze, 2009, 524 - 25).

In: Nerve Sheath Tumors
Editor: Richard A. Prayson

ISBN: 978-1-53617-366-6
© 2020 Nova Science Publishers, Inc.

Chapter 3

PERIPHERAL NERVE SHEATH TUMORS OF THE ORAL CAVITY AND JAW

Bryan B. Hair[1] and Richard A. Prayson, MD, MEd[*]
Cleveland Clinic Lerner College of Medicine of Case Western Reserve University School of Medicine and
Cleveland Clinic Department of Anatomic Pathology
Cleveland Clinic Foundation, Cleveland, OH, US

ABSTRACT

Peripheral nerve sheath tumors of the oral cavity and jaw are rare entities with limited discussion in the literature. There are both benign and malignant tumor subtypes, and although they all derive from nerves or other cells of the neural sheath, their histology, clinical behavior, and preferred treatment strategies are distinct. The following subtypes are included in this chapter: schwannoma, neurofibroma, palisaded encapsulated neuroma, perineurioma, mucosal neuroma, nerve sheath myxoma, granular cell tumor, and malignant peripheral nerve sheath tumor. Traumatic neuroma, though not a true neoplasm, is also included.

---

[1] Bryan B Hair, BS.
[*] Corresponding Author's Email: praysor@ccf.org; Fax: 216-445-6967.

These neoplasms can occur at disparate locations within the oral cavity such as the submandibular triangle, mandible, palate, lips, oral mucosa, and tongue. Many features are thought to be similar to peripheral nerve sheath tumors of other primary locations, though there are important differences. The differential diagnosis is also distinct for lesions encountered in the oral cavity. Some of the aforementioned tumor types are associated with syndromes such as neurofibromatosis type 1 and multiple endocrine neoplasia type IIB, and there are clinically relevant distinctions between patients with syndromic rather than sporadic tumors. This chapter will consolidate our understanding of this uncommon yet clinically significant tumor category as it relates to epidemiology, tumor etiology, clinical presentation, histopathological characteristics, diagnosis, treatment, and patient outcomes.

INTRODUCTION

Neurogenic tumors of the oral cavity and jaw comprise rare and heterogeneous neoplasms that, as do all peripheral nerve sheath tumors (PNSTs), arise from perineurial cells, myelin producing Schwann cells, connective tissue within nerves, or other components of the epineurium or perineurium [1]. Though the majority of peripheral nerve sheath tumors are inherently benign, there are cases of highly aggressive, de novo malignant neoplasms in addition to the malignant transformation of benign tumors [2]. Historically, the major subtypes of benign PNST include schwannoma, traumatic neuroma, neurofibroma, palisaded encapsulated neuroma, perineurioma, mucosal neuroma, nerve sheath myxoma, and granular cell tumor. All malignant lesions are now grouped in to a single category referred to as malignant peripheral nerve sheath tumors (MPNSTs). A separate category of PNST labeled hybrid PNST, comprises tumors that exhibit intermixed components of schwannoma, neurofibroma, and perineurioma, and this rare but unique entity is not discussed in this chapter [3].

Because nerve sheath tumors of the jaw and oral cavity are exceedingly rare, there is a dearth of information in the current literature regarding their epidemiology, etiology, clinical presentation, histopathological characteristics, diagnosis, treatment, and outcomes. This chapter will attempt to consolidate the information that is currently available as it relates to the aforementioned topics.

The epidemiological data regarding PNSTs of the oral cavity and jaw is very limited. A seminal study on solitary peripheral nerve tumors found that 45% of these arose in the head and neck, and of these, 22% originated in the oral cavity [4, 5]. A more recent retrospective study found that PNSTs were only encountered in 0.2% of all biopsied lesions in the oral cavity and almost half of these were classified as traumatic neuromas [6]. There are only individual case reports of malignant intraoral PNSTs and roughly 50% of them are believed to have occurred in individuals with comorbid neurofibromatosis type I [7]. The epidemiological data for each neoplasm will be discussed in context within the sections that follow.

MALIGNANT PERIPHERAL NERVE SHEATH TUMOR

This heterogeneous group of malignant tumors was previously referred to with labels such as neurogenic sarcoma, neurilemmosarcoma, malignant fibrosarcoma and malignant neurilemmoma up until the early 1990s when MPNST became the preferred term [8, 9]. The World Health Organization acknowledged this updated categorization and subsequently designated MPNST as a soft-tissue sarcoma [10, 11]. As of 2016, two subtypes are officially recognized: epithelioid MPNST and MPNST with perineurial differentiation. Other variants such as malignant Triton tumor and glandular MPNST are considered to be histological patterns of MPNST [12]. Although MPNSTs share similar biological and clinical features, in reality, they represent multiple entities with varied cellular differentiation, cytogenetic characteristics, and histological patterns. This fact, in combination with a general lack of standardized or unique diagnostic features, makes MPNSTs notoriously difficult to diagnose and distinguish from benign PNSTs and other spindle cell sarcomas [13, 14].

Etiology

The term malignant peripheral nerve sheath tumor (MPNST) encompass all malignant neoplasms that arise from the nerve sheath with the exception of epineurial, vascular, and inflammatory cells. This category also includes malignant neoplasms that exhibit Schwann or perineurial cell differentiation, even if the tumor itself is unassociated with a nerve [15]. MPNST does not include tumors that arise for the epineurium or from the vasculature within nerves. Similarly, malignant granular cell tumors, which will be discussed later in this chapter, are also excluded from this category [7].

The molecular and genetic etiological factors in MPNST have received considerable study but are yet to be fully elucidated. This subject will be discussed only briefly here. For clarity, the specific clinical and epidemiological information related to the malignant transformation of benign entities is discussed in the context of the each of the PNST subtypes that are covered later in this chapter.

The loss of the tumor suppressor NF1 gene is clearly an important predisposing factor for the development of MPNST, but additional molecular and genetic changes are required to ultimately drive the neoplastic process. There are various non-syndromic cases of MPNST that do not exhibit loss of NF1; thus, there is continued debate on whether or not NF1 loss is truly a ubiquitous oncogenic feature [16]. Recent genomic studies have implicated additional genes and proteins in the neoplastic process. Those with the greatest association include SUZ12, EED, TP53, p16 (INK4A), CDKN2A, c-Kit, EGFR, c-Met, and platelet-derived growth factor-α. Many of these, such as SUZ12 and EED, code for proteins involved in a complex that modulates the RAS signaling cascade [16-18]. Therefore, mutations in these genes can result in disinhibited RAS activation. NF1 mutations have similarly been demonstrated to increase RAS activation. There is some evidence, particularly in non-syndromic individuals, that BRAF V600E mutations can yield similar molecular consequences [17].

At a gross genomic level, MPNSTs have complex karyotypes with an average 18 aberrations per tumor with significant intra and intertumoral heterogeneity. Common irregularities include large deletions on chromosomes 1p, 9p, 11q, 12p, 13q, 14q, 17p 18, 22q, X, and Y, with focal gains on chromosomes 7, 8q, 15q and 17q [7, 16]. No consistent translocations are observed in MPNSTs.

Epidemiology

It is estimated that as many as 50% of all MPNSTs occur in patients with NF1 and the lifetime risk for these individuals is between 2-5 percent [19, 20]. This risk can be further stratified as those with symptomatic plexiform neurofibromas or large genetic rearrangements in the NF1 gene have much higher risk than those that do not [20]. One in ten MPNSTs are associated with prior radiation exposure [21]. Overall, MPNSTs are rare and account for approximately 5-10% of soft tissue sarcomas, which have an overall incidence that is estimated to be 5 people per million per year [22, 23]. No difference in male or female incidence has been demonstrated for sporadic cases but there is a greater prevalence of male NF1 patients (and therefore more MPNSTs) [13, 24]. The oral cavity is an uncommon anatomical site for MPNSTs (only one in nine affect the head and neck) and only a small percentage arise there. Nevertheless, the most common intra-oral subsites of MPNST include the tongue and soft palate though involvement of the mandible, lip, and buccal mucosa have been reported as well [21]. Most cases of de novo MPNST occur in the 2nd to 5th decades of life; whereas, they tend to occur even earlier in individuals with NF1 [19]. The small number of oral MPNSTs described in the literature are consistent with the above epidemiology for anatomically nonspecific MPNSTs [25].

Clinical Presentation and Diagnosis

Clinically, MPNSTs classically present as a slow growing mass or fullness with occasional concomitant pain (more frequent in patients with

NF1). Additional symptoms can include paresthesia, weakness, or changes to an already existing mass or lesion [20]. In a majority of cases, the mass is greater than 5 cm at the time of presentation and oral lesions are described as flesh-colored, submucosal, well-circumscribed, sessile, and bosselated [21]. In general, they appear similar to other soft tissue neoplasms and sectioning commonly reveals necrosis and/or hemorrhage [13]. They are highly aggressive neoplasms and as many as 50% of patients are thought to have metastatic disease at the time of presentation; therefore, a thorough physical exam and radiologic evaluation are essential in identifying sites of potential distant metastasis. Lung examination and computed tomography (CT) of the chest and/or positron emission tomography (PET) are of particular importance in order to rule out distant metastasis [7]. Interestingly, of the 17 cases of confirmed intraoral MPNST documented in the literature since 1973, only one had documented distant metastasis (pelvis) [23]. Preoperatively, magnetic resonance imaging (MRI) is the modality of choice for imaging of the primary mass, although in many cases, surgeons forego this imaging when the mass can be visualized and palpated on exam [23].

In general, sarcomas are assumed to be MPNSTs if at least one of the following three criteria are met:

> "(1) the tumor arises from a peripheral nerve and shows no aberrant or heterologous line of differentiation; (2) it arises from a preexisting benign nerve sheath tumor, usually a neurofibroma; or (3) the tumor displays a constellation of histologic features that are seen in tumors arising in the foregoing situations and are considered typical of malignant Schwann cell tumors" (described below) [7, 20].

While these criteria are helpful for establishing the diagnosis of MPNST in many cases, exceptions are common and histologic aberrations and challenges are included in the discussion that follows.

Pathology and Immunohistochemistry

Histologically, MPNSTs most often display fascicles of monotonous spindle cells that are woven into a herringbone pattern with enlarged and hyperchromatic nuclei that may resemble those of a typical Schwann cell. At low magnification, distinct areas of low and high cellularity may be visualized [7]. Other subtle features of nerve sheath differentiation may be apparent, such as nuclear palisading and perivascular whirling. Cellular pleomorphism, mitotic activity, and necrosis are also common (Figures 1-3) [1]. It is not always possible to identify a peripheral nerve or parent lesion from which the tumor originates. Elements of bone, cartilage, glands and muscle differentiation can be observed, which can further complicate the diagnosis [9, 26]. The aforementioned differentiation patterns may portend a worse prognosis and almost all MPNSTs are graded as intermediate to high [7]. Some authors describe the herniation of tumor into blood vessels which results in small vessels proliferating within the walls of larger blood vessels as another subtle feature that may be indicative of MPNST [13].

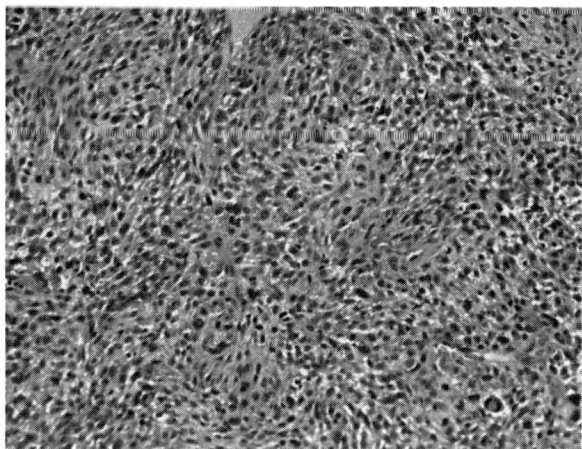

Figure 1. Malignant peripheral nerve sheath tumor marked by prominent hypercellularity and nuclear atypia (hematoxylin and eosin, original magnification 200X).

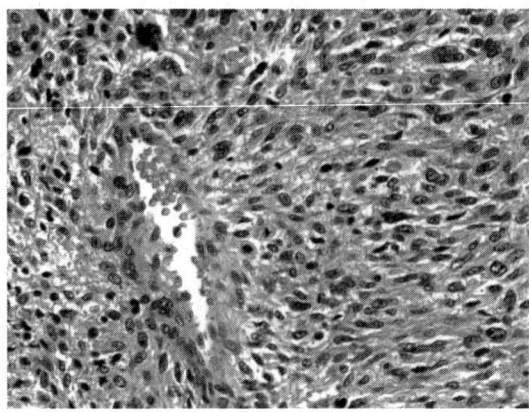

Figure 2. Mitotic figures are frequently encountered in malignant peripheral nerve sheath tumors (hematoxylin and eosin, original magnification 400X).

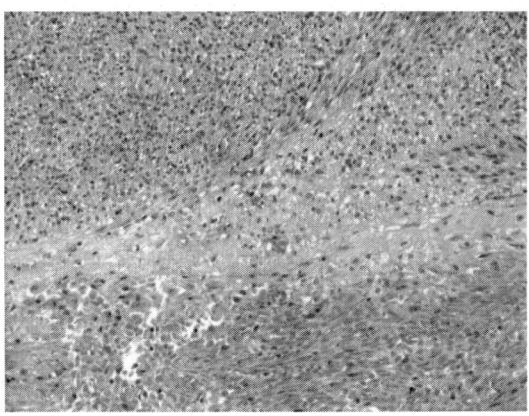

Figure 3. Malignant peripheral nerve sheath tumors often are marked by geographic areas of necrosis (bottom) (hematoxylin and eosin, original magnification 200X).

MPNSTs stain positively for S-100 protein in approximately 50% of cases. It is reported that other markers such as vimentin, CD56, EMA, myelin basic protein, SOX-10, p75, Ki-67, Leu-7, nestin, H3K27me3, and PGP9.5 may be suggestive of MPNST but are variable and cannot be used reliably for diagnosis [27-29]. Unfortunately as of yet, there remains no definitive genetic or molecular biomarker for the diagnosis of MPNST as all are nonspecific and observed in a variety of benign and malignant lesions [18].

Treatment and Outcomes

Definitive local surgery with negative margins is the preferred treatment approach for qualifying patients with localized lesions of the oral cavity. The risk of lymphatic spread with MPNST is low and thus neck dissection is seldom recommended at the time of primary extirpation [23]. Hematogenous spread and perineural invasion/extension are common [30]. If a major nerve is observed intraoperatively to be grossly invaded by the sarcoma, it is critical to obtain proximal nerve specimens for frozen histological analysis until negative margins are obtained. Local recurrence rates following definitive local treatment are 40-42% within the first postoperative year [7, 23]. Overall, prognosis is poor and the 5-year survival rate is between 40 and 75%. There is limited evidence that the prognosis is worse for patients with NF1 as opposed to sporadic tumors [21]. Adjuvant radiation is recommended for large primary tumors or those with high risk features to prevent local recurrence. Adjuvant chemotherapy for soft tissue carcinomas in general has shown marginal survival benefits, though there is no evidence to specifically support benefit to patients with MPNST; it can therefore be considered as a treatment option in select cases [7]. Chemotherapy for distant disease has shown a response rate of approximately 21% and outcomes remain extremely poor. There are various ongoing studies and clinical trials exploring possible targeted therapies [7].

SCHWANNOMA

Etiology

Schwannomas are benign neoplasms that arise from Schwann cells. A seminal population-based study suggested that 90% occur sporadically with the remainder occurring in relation to NF1, NF2, Carney's complex, or schwannomatosis [31]. Loss of the tumor suppressor protein merlin (product of the NF2 gene) is a shared molecular factor in both the syndromic and sporadic cases. As such, mutations or complete loss of chromosome 22q are common cytogenetic features of schwannoma [2, 31]. Various other differences in cytogenetics and gene expression have been reported though their roles in disease pathogenesis remain unclear.

Epidemiology

Intraoral schwannomas are documented to occur at similar rates between men and women and the most frequent anatomic location is the tongue (about 50% of cases) [32]. Other less frequent locations include the palate, floor of mouth, buccal mucosa, gingiva, lips, and vestibular mucosa [5, 32]. As of 2010, 46 intraosseous schwannomas had been confirmed in the literature with 85% occurring in the mandible and 15% occurring in the maxilla [33]. The peak prevalence occurs in the second to third decades of life, similar to other peripheral schwannomas [34–36].

Clinical Presentation and Diagnosis

Schwannomas are slow growing and fully encapsulated by the epineurium. Grossly, they are typically less than 5 cm in diameter with a soft tan-white appearance [37]. Identification of a painless mass or swelling is the most common presenting symptom, followed by symptomatic sequelae related to nerve compression (such as pain, paresthesia, numbness, etc.) [38]. Intraosseous schwannomas are usually asymptomatic and are frequently diagnosed incidentally [33].

Pathology and Immunohistochemistry

Schwannomas are inherently low-grade (World Health Organization (WHO) grade I) and histologically diverse. Conventional schwannomas are comprised of spindle cells with an absence of axons within the tumor proper. It is frequently observed that axons and perineurial cells are aggregated to the periphery of the mass [31]. Microscopically, the tissue architecture is biphasic and contains compact and loose cellular regions, termed Antoni A and Antoni B areas, respectively. In Antoni A areas, the cells are arranged in bundles and interlacing fascicles and the individual cells have twisted nuclei with occasional intranuclear vacuoles and poorly defined cytoplasmic borders. Antoni B areas, on the other hand, are more disorganized with markedly less cellularity. Spindle cells are dispersed in a background matrix that is interspersed with collagen, inflammatory cells, microcystic changes, and irregularly spaced blood vessels (Figure 4) [2]. Verocay bodies, or areas of nuclear palisading around acellular areas are often encountered in Antoni A areas and are pathognomonic for schwannoma (Figure 5) [5]. The ratio between Antoni A and Antoni B areas is unpredictable but the former tends to predominate within intraoral schwannomas [2, 39]. Large tumors often exhibit degenerative changes such as cyst formation, aggregation of lipid-laden macrophages, and clusters of hyalinized blood vessels that can thrombose and result in hemosiderin-laden macrophages. When regions of large and atypical hyperchromatic nuclei are observed, this is referred to as "ancient change" and has been described in the oral cavity. Care should be taken to not conflate ancient change with true malignant transformation [31, 40]. In a minority of specimens, giant rosettes formed by small lymphocyte-like Schwann cells that are organized around collagen nodules or blood vessels are described [2].

Immunohistochemically, almost all of the tumor cells have the antigenic phenotype of a classic Schwann cell including abundant S-100 protein; staining for SOX10, a well-characterized intranuclear marker of neural crest differentiation, is also useful diagnostically [2]. The majority of schwannomas are also positive for GFAP, Leu-7, and CD34/EPA staining (CD34 is positive in the capsule) [41]. Immunohistochemical studies are particularly important in cases where tumor degeneration, fibrosis, or myxoid change obscure the natural histology and thus preclude confident histologically-based diagnosis. It can also be used to rule out tumors with similar histologic features such as leiomyosarcoma [2].

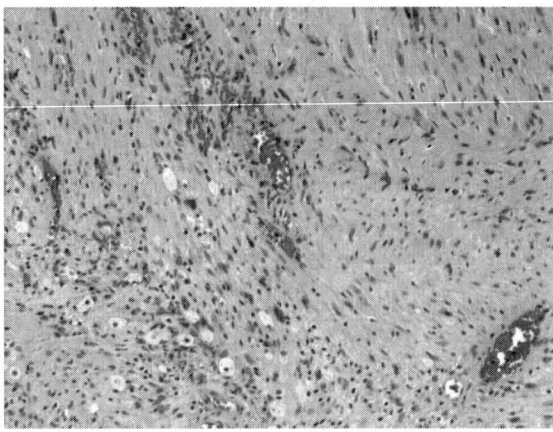

Figure 4. Schwannomas are marked by a proliferation of spindled cells with tapered nuclei. Some tumors demonstrate nuclear pleomorphism and contain macrophages, as seen in this tumor (hematoxylin and eosin, original magnification 200X).

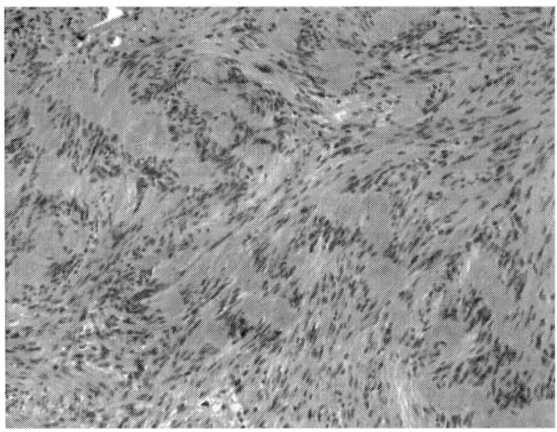

Figure 5. Palisaded nuclei characterize the Verocay body, a fairly characteristic although not invariably present feature of schwannomas (hematoxylin and eosin, original magnification 200X).

Treatment and Outcomes

Surgical resection is the treatment of choice with preservation of the nerve, if possible. In many cases, the tumor can be readily dissected from the nerve, though in some cases, sacrifice may be necessary. Radiotherapy can be considered for patients who are not good surgical candidates. Recurrence is rare and morbidity and mortality are low. There are documented cases of malignant transformation of intraoral schwannomas, though this is exceptionally rare and a subject of controversy [38, 42].

TRAUMATIC NEUROMA

Etiology

Traumatic neuromas are hyperplastic lesions comprised of Schwann cells and regenerating axons and they do not constitute a true neoplastic entity. Damage to the nerve, most frequently through injury or surgery, is the initial causal mechanism and can occur in peripheral somatic, autonomic, and cranial nerves [43, 44]. The proliferative process is initiated in the proximal axon in response to Wallerian degeneration of the distal nerve [45]. Physiologic repair is possible when there is continuity or close apposition of nerves at the site of damage. When repair is unsuccessful, the regenerative process can become disorganized and result in the formation of a traumatic neuroma [2]. As such, a thorough clinical history is paramount, when clinically evaluating a potential traumatic neuroma.

Epidemiology

Traumatic neuromas, as the name implies, occur secondary to injury or surgery and thus have no natural age predilection. Epidemiological data regarding the incidence of intraoral traumatic neuromas is sparse, but prospectively collected single-institution data suggests that they account for 6.2% of benign, pathologically diagnosed tumors in the oral cavity and 0.34% of all oral pathologic diagnoses [46]. They also found that there was a 1.85 female to male ratio [46]. The anatomical sites most frequently involved (in descending order) include the mental foramen, lower lip, tongue, buccal mucosa, hard palate, posterior mandible, canine fossa, and maxillary anterior ridge [47]. In general, the inferior alveolar nerve is more frequently affected than the lingual nerve [44, 47].

Clinical Presentation and Diagnosis

Most traumatic neuromas are asymptomatic; nevertheless, a minority result in acute and chronic pain. The exact etiology of the pain remains unclear but may involve strangulation of tissue, local trauma, or infection [2]. Grossly, they are usually less than two centimeters in length and appear as firm ovular nodules but can be variable in shape. Traumatic neuromas are not encapsulated. The lesion itself is usually embedded in surrounding scar tissue [43]. A biopsy to confirm the diagnosis of traumatic neuroma may be necessary, especially in patients with a history of head and neck cancer, in order to rule out the possibility of oncologic recurrence.

Pathology and Immunohistochemistry

A disorganized proliferation of nerve fascicles with accompanying Schwann cells and fibroblasts within a moderately loose fibrovascular stroma characterizes the standard histologic appearance of the traumatic neuroma (Figure 6) [2]. The axons within this hyperplastic lesion exhibit inconsistent and unpredictable patterns of myelination. The mass is always identified at the end of a damaged nerve and evidence of Wallerian degeneration may be observed in the parent nerve, if the lesion is relatively new [21]. Irritation fibromas may morphologically resemble a nerve sheath tumor or traumatic neuroma; they are marked by spindled fibroblasts with intervening collagen (Figure 7).

The immunohistochemical profile described is consistent with what would be expected, granted the various cell types present within the hyperplastic lesion. The literature documents that traumatic neuromas are S-

100 positive, Leu-7 positive (weak), EMA positive (perineurium), and CD34 positive (weak) [29].

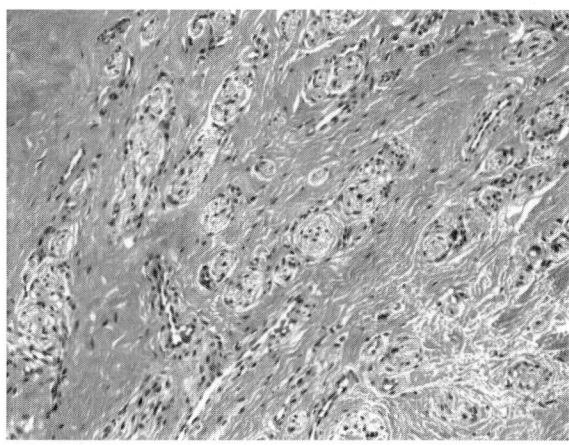

Figure 6. A traumatic neuroma is marked by small bundles of disorganized peripheral nerve tissue intermixed with collagen (hematoxylin and eosin, original magnification 200X).

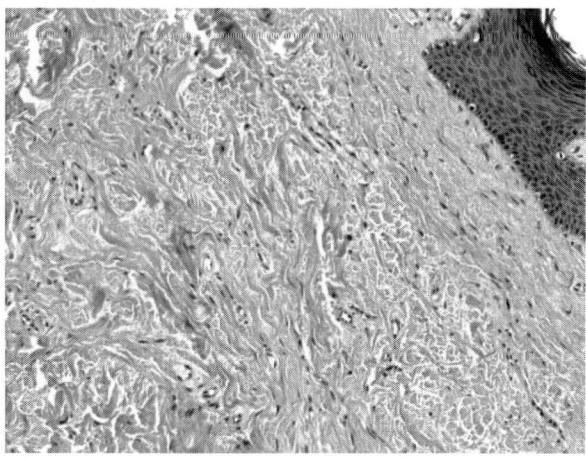

Figure 7. Irritation fibromas can at times mimic peripheral nerve sheath tumors; they are comprised of spindled cells (fibroblasts) with intervening collagen (hematoxylin and eosin, original magnification 200X).

Treatment and Outcomes

Surgical resection is the definitive treatment but this is only indicated if the patient experiences symptoms that have a significant effect on their quality of life. During the procedure, the hyperplastic mass is removed and end of the nerve is repositioned into another location [2]. Pharmacotherapy with analgesics, NMDA receptor antagonists, antidepressants, and anticonvulsants have been utilized for symptomatic relief in addition to other conservative approaches such as physical therapy, direct nerve stimulation, and acupuncture [45]. Traumatic neuromas have no malignant potential and post-excisional recurrence is rare [48].

NEUROFIBROMA

Etiology

The cell type from which neurofibromas arise continues to be disputed in the literature. There is evidence to support an origin from Schwann cells, endoneurial fibroblasts, perineurial cells, or an intermediate between these cell types [49]. Neurofibromas can be classified based on their patterns of growth and whether or not they arise from a single peripheral nerve or from multiple nerve bundles. These are referred to as myxoid (dermal) and plexiform neurofibromas, respectively. The third type is diffuse neurofibroma, which is characterized by an ill-defined mass that extends along adipose and connective tissue and surrounds non-involved structures [2, 50]. Neurofibromas can also be classified into major and minor tumor subtypes based on their morphological features [51]. All neurofibromas arise from defects in the NF1 gene on chromosome 17 in accordance with the Knudson two-hit hypothesis [52].

Epidemiology

Neurofibromas are often dichotomized into those that occur in relation to NF1 and those that occur as solitary (non-syndromic) lesions. Roughly, 6.5% of all solitary neurofibromas occur in the oral cavity and this percentage is thought to be greater in NF1 [53, 54]. Current evidence suggests that the majority of solitary neurofibromas occur idiopathically; whereas, a minority are syndromic [2, 55]. Accurate estimates are precluded by the difficult and often delayed diagnosis of NF1. Multiple synchronous lesions and plexiform lesions of the oral cavity occur less frequently and are associated with neurofibromatosis to a greater extent [49]. Both sexes are thought to be affected similarly and the most common age of diagnosis of solitary neurofibromas is in the 3rd decade [21, 56, 57]. Data suggests that patients with NF1 present earlier, on average, and over 80% develop a neurofibroma prior to the age of 30 years [58]. The tongue, buccal mucosa, and vestibular areas are the most common sites, although additional locations such as the palate, cheek mucosa, floor of the mouth, and intraosseous sites have been reported as well [5, 26]. Single-institution data suggests that 7.7% of all benign oral tumors and 0.43% of all oral biopsies were diagnosed as neurofibroma [46].

Clinical Presentation and Diagnosis

Oral neurofibromas are circumscribed but non-encapsulated slow growing tumors that can present as sessile mobile masses that involve the surface mucosa [50]. The tumor itself is often described as a gray-tan, glossy, and homogenous in nature [59]. Plexiform neurofibromas are classically described as having the appearance of a "bag of worms" and generally cause more extensive disfigurement and morbidity [50]. Overall, tumors of the oral cavity show similar characteristics to those found elsewhere in the body although there is often no distinct border between the tumor and the surrounding tissue [26]. Clinically, neurofibromas follow an indolent course and only rarely present with pain, pruritus, or paresthesia.

The diagnosis must be confirmed via pathology, either with biopsy or complete resection [21]. Patients presenting with confirmed neurofibromas should be evaluated for the diagnosis of NF1, especially if they present with multiple or plexiform neurofibromas.

Pathology and Immunohistochemistry

Microscopically, neurofibromas exhibit loose and disorganized spindle cells of mild to moderate cellularity in a background matrix composed primarily by collagen (Figure 8). The cells are described as having bent or wavy nuclei that are sometimes described as having a "diving dolphin" appearance. Mast cells are commonly found within the tumor [55]. Tactile corpuscle-like structures referred to as Wagner Meissner bodies may be encountered (Figure 9).

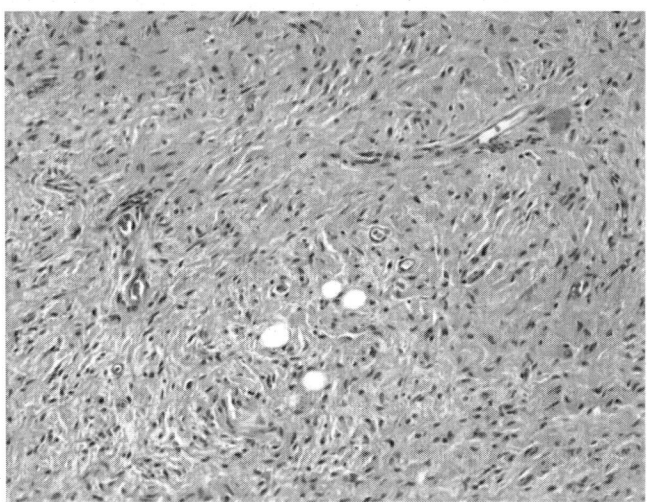

Figure 8. Bland spindled cells spaced apart from one another characterizes a neurofibroma (hematoxylin and eosin, original magnification 200X).

Neurofibromas stain positively for S-100 (approximately 50% of tumor cells), EMA (to a small extent in perineural cells), and myelin basic protein. They also stain positively for CD34 in a distinct fashion described in the literature as "fingerprint immunopositivity" (as the staining between the whorled collagen bundles produces a distinct pattern that is pathognomonic for neurofibroma) [55].

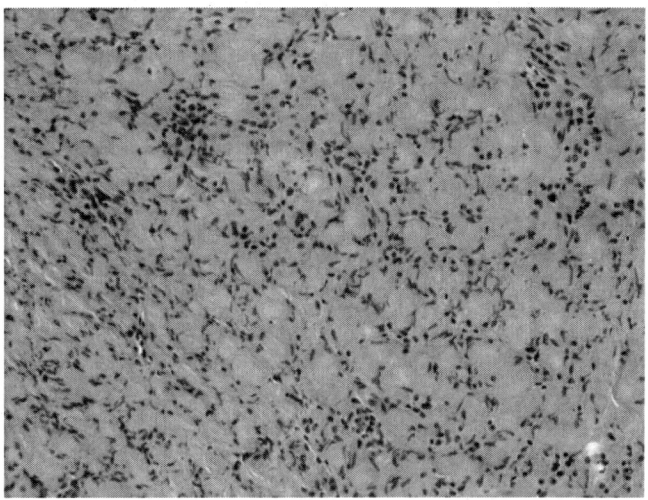

Figure 9. Tactile corpuscle-like bodies known as Wagner Meissner bodies in a neurofibroma (hematoxylin and eosin, original magnification 200X).

Treatment and Outcomes

Surgical resection is the recommended treatment in select cases with functional and/or cosmetic complaints. Dissection of the tumor from the nerve is often difficult to accomplish, as the two structures can be closely intertwined [50]. Spontaneous resolution of the tumor following puberty has been reported and thus some clinicians recommend surveillance as a viable option for pediatric patients with solitary lesions [59]. Recurrence following surgical excision is extremely rare though perhaps slightly more common in the head and neck; nevertheless, there is some evidence that recurrence portends an increased risk of malignant transformation [53,57]. Malignant transformation of non-syndromic solitary nodules is extremely rare and possibly even non-existent. In persons with NF1, epidemiological studies have found a 10-12% lifetime risk of malignant transformation. When transformation does occur, neurofibrosarcoma and malignant neurilemmoma (malignant schwannoma) are the most common pathologies [21]. Interestingly, malignant transformation is disproportionately uncommon in the head and neck, and even more so in the oral cavity [60].

PALISADED ENCAPSULATED NEUROMA

Etiology

Palisaded encapsulated neuromas (PEN) were only identified as a discrete tumor class in 1972, as they share many characteristics with schwannomas [2, 61, 62]. Similar to traumatic neuromas, PENs represent hyperplasia as opposed to a true neoplastic process and are thought to result from nerve damage or local inflammation [61]. The growth is created secondary to the proliferation of Schwann cells in an aligned and occasionally palisaded pattern. They differ from schwannomas in that axons are interspersed within the tumor and there is generally a lack of stromal change commonly observed in other tumor types. They are either completely or partially encapsulated by the perineurium, and as with neurofibromas, there are distinct morphological patterns observed clinically. Plexiform, vascular, myxoid, epithelioid, fungating, and multinodular PENs have all been described in the literature [61].

Epidemiology

PENs, sometimes referred to as solitary circumscribed neuromas, most commonly affect the skin and mucosal tissue. Anatomically, the masticatory mucosa (palate and gingiva) is involved, most frequently followed by the labial, tongue, and buccal mucosa [61]. Both sexes are equally affected and diagnosis is most common in the 5th to 7th decade of life [62]. Single-institution data suggests that 0.05% of oral biopsies were read as PEN [63].

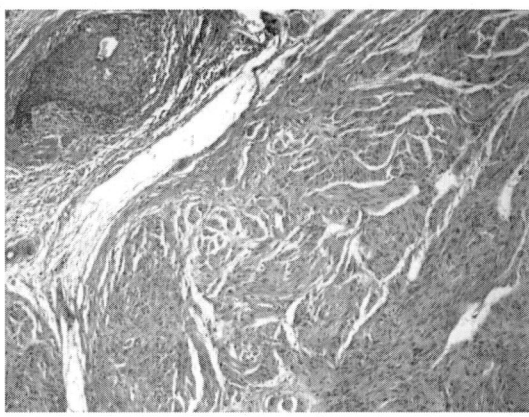

Figure 10. A palisaded encapsulated neuroma marked by spindled cells arranged in vague fascicles and cellular whorling (hematoxylin and eosin, original magnification 100X).

Clinical Presentation and Diagnosis

PENs are described as well circumscribed, small, slow growing, nodular, firm, and non-pigmented masses that are almost always asymptomatic [62]. They almost always occur as solitary masses; there are rare cases of multiple synchronous PENs, but this is yet to be reported in the oral cavity [64]. The diagnosis must be confirmed via pathology either with biopsy or complete resection.

Pathology and Immunohistochemistry

Microscopically, PENs are moderately cellular and proliferative Schwann cells are observed to form fascicles or microfascicles that are disorganized in nature (Figure 10). There are sometimes small clefts and limited myxoid areas separating these structures [65]. The cell nuclei appear elongated, wavy, and oval shaped with occasional nuclear holes (Lockhern change) [21, 61]. It is not uncommon for oral PENs to have focal areas of nuclear palisading that appear similar to Verocay bodies, and these can be indistinguishable from those of schwannomas. Nevertheless, because many PENs lack this feature, the name solitary circumscribed neuroma (SCN) is felt by many to be a more appropriate name [21]. Nuclear atypia, pleomorphism, and mitotic activity are very rarely observed in these tumors. The tumors generally contain few capillaries though there are cases of vascular variants in the literature [61]. As with neurofibroma, infrequent mast cells can be observed in PEN [62]. Though overlying mucosal changes such as acanthosis, basal cell hyperplasia, and pseudoepitheliomatous hyperplasia have been encountered, oral PENs most frequently exhibit mucosal atrophy [61].

The tumor cells within PENs stain positively for S-100 protein (with rare S-100 negative fibroblasts) and vimentin but negatively for GFAP, which can be useful (in addition to staining for axons) in distinguishing PEN from schwannoma, when Verocay bodies are present [2,61]. The perineurial envelope is readily observed with EMA, Claudin-1 or GLUT-1 immunostains. Weak CD34 positivity is also reported in the literature [41].

Treatment and Outcomes

Conservative local excision is the preferred treatment as there is minimal risk of recurrence and transformation. In a review of 55 cases, recurrence was only documented in a single case [61, 66]. Laser ablation is also described in the literature [64]. This type of PNST is not associated with any known hereditary syndromes; therefore, genetic screening and oncologic surveillance are not required.

PERINEURIOMA

Etiology

Perineurioma is a benign neoplasm comprised of cells that demonstrate advanced perineurial differentiation [67]. It was first described in 1978 and several subtypes have since been defined, including intraneural, extraneural (formerly known as storiform perineurial fibroma), sclerosing, mucosal, and reticular [2, 68]. Deletions of 22q and other point mutations of the NF2 gene are commonly observed in perineuriomas; nevertheless, this feature is not ubiquitous and perineuriomas are not associated with neurofibromatosis. There continues to be some debate on whether the process is reactive or truly neoplastic and some researchers consider perineurioma to be the peripheral counterpart to meningioma [67, 68, 69].

Epidemiology

Perineurioma is an uncommon PNST and it is exceedingly rare for it to occur in the oral cavity or jaw. Soft tissue (extraneural) perineuriomas present most frequently in middle age (with a large standard deviation) and there is no documented gender predominance [68]. Conversely, intraneural and sclerosing perineuriomas classically present in young adulthood (also no gender predominance) [68]. As of 2019, there are 22 documented cases of intraoral extraneural perineurioma and 17 cases of intranueral perineurioma [69, 70]

Clinical Presentation and Diagnosis

Because intraneural perineuriomas originate within a peripheral nerve sheath, it is common for patients to present clinically with symptoms such as pain, paresthesia, numbness, or motor deficits related to nerve compression [70]. Extraneural perineuriomas, on the other hand, almost always present asymptomatically. In both cases, perineuriomas of the oral cavity have been described as indolent, small, well-circumscribed, white or tan, and painless nodules. Intraneural perineuriomas are often described as multinodular fusiform outgrowths from nerves [67]. Perineuriomas can share many histological similarities to neurofibroma, schwannoma, and fibrous histiocytoma and thus correlation with immunohistochemical findings is often necessary for diagnosis [70].

Pathology and Immunohistochemistry

Microscopically, perineuriomas are described as having a whorled, storiform, and lamellar growth patterns with varied cellularity [68]. As with many other spindle cell neoplasms, the cells are narrow with wavy nuclei in a background of collagenous or myxoid stroma (Figure 11). Cellular pleomorphism or focally invasive margins are sometimes described but these findings carry no known clinical significance [67]. The spindle cells of intraneural perineuriomas are observed to surround individual axons and Schwann cells resulting in the formation of "onion-bulb" like structures on cross section [68].

Immunohistochemically, EMA is an important marker that is positive in almost all cases of perineurioma (Figure 12). Other markers, including GLUT-1, claudin, and CD34 often stain the tumor positively but they have poor sensitivity and are nonspecific. S-100 protein is seldom present in perineuriomas, especially those that are extraneural [68]. Some research suggests that staining for somatostatin receptor 2 and progesterone receptor can help to differentiate perineuriomas from the very rare extra-cranial meningioma [70].

Treatment and Outcomes

Perineuriomas are benign and simple excision is sufficient when clinically indicated [68]. There is only one documented case of (potential) local recurrence of perineurioma in the oral cavity. There is a rare subtype of MPNST, sometimes referred to as malignant perineurioma, that exhibits perineurial differentiation but malignant transformation from a perineurioma remains undocumented in the literature [71, 72].

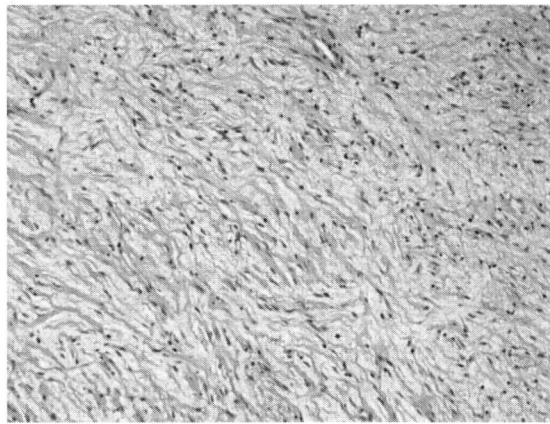

Figure 11. A perineurioma marked by bland spindled cells arranged against a myxoid stroma (hematoxylin and eosin, original magnification 200X).

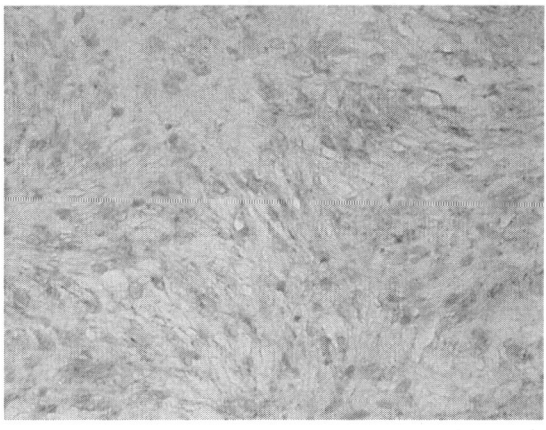

Figure 12. Perineurioma demonstrating epithelial membrane antigen (EMA) positivity (original magnification 400X).

MUCOSAL NEUROMA

Etiology

Mucosal neuromas (MNs) are of neuroendocrine origin, and in most cases, are associated with mutations in the RET proto-oncogene and multiple endocrine neoplasia type IIB (MEN IIB) (otherwise referred to as MEN III or mucosal neuroma syndrome) [21, 73]. There is only a single genetically validated case that describes oral mucosal neuromas in a patient in which the diagnosis of MEN IIB was definitively ruled out, thus providing some evidence that a minor or variant form of this condition may exist [74,75]

Epidemiology

MNs are a cardinal and distinguishing feature of multiple endocrine neoplasia type IIB, though there exist individual case reports that document oral mucosal neuromas in patients that were confirmed to not have MEN IIB [76]. The prevalence of MEN IIB is estimated to be between 1 in 600,000 and 1 in 4 million and both sexes are affected equally [77]. MNs usually manifest shortly after birth as opposed to the associated adrenal and thyroid tumors which manifest later in life [21, 78].

Clinical Presentation and Diagnosis

Clinically, they most frequently present as multiple yellow-white painless papules or pedunculated nodules of the tongue that are less than 1 centimeter in diameter [21, 74]. The mass is found in the submucosa, is partially encapsulated, and comprised of irregular and tortuous nerve bundles within a prominent perineurium [2, 21]. Persons should be screened appropriately for MEN IIB and followed up in accordance with the standard of care for this population (if positive).

Pathology and Immunohistochemistry

MNs arise in the submucosa and consist of irregular and tortuously entangled nerve bundles within an enlarged perineurium. These features distinguish many MNs from histologically similar traumatic neuromas [21].

There is often prominent myxoid change within a background of loose fibrous stroma. Inflammatory cells and dysplasia are not typically observed [2]. The nerves themselves appear histologically normal but may demonstrate focal areas of hyperplasia or bulbous expansion [21].

The immunohistochemical profile of MNs describes positive staining for S-100 protein, collagen type IV, vimentin, neuron specific enolase, and neurofilament. Some masses with greater perineurial differentiation also stain positively for EMA [21]

Treatment and Outcomes

Treatment via surgical excision is reserved for cases with functional and/or aesthetic complaints. These lesions are considered to be invariably benign with no malignant potential though nearly 50% recur [2]

NERVE SHEATH MYXOMA

Etiology

Nerve sheath myxoma (NSM) was first described in 1969 and has been canonically subcategorized as either classical, cellular, or mixed based on the quantity of myxoid stroma [79]. Neurothekeomas share many characteristics with NSM and since their discovery in 1980, many authors aberrantly considered them to be variants of the same tumor (as such, the terms are often erroneously used synonymously in the literature). It is now generally acknowledged that they are indeed distinct entities with unique cellular origins and features [79]. Differential gene expression likewise supports this view [2]. There continues to exist controversy on whether or not the cellular and mixed subtypes both truly derive from a neural origin. There is some evidence to suggest that all NSMs and neurothekeomas exist within a spectrum (and all demonstrate neural differentiation, at least to an extent) and this may signify that they indeed share a common origin from a neural cellular lineage [80]. In many of the oral case reports, there is a history of trauma in the area, possibly implicating tissue damage as an etiological factor.

Epidemiology

There are currently only 28 cases of intraoral nerve sheath myxoma, (including cases in which they were referred to as neurothekoma) in the literature. The gender ratio is close to 1:1 and there is a wide range in the age of diagnosis. The most common intraoral site is the tongue followed by the buccal mucosa, palate, and lower lip [81, 82].

Clinical Presentation and Diagnosis

NSM of the oral cavity has been described as a slow growing and elastic lobular mass that is, on average, 1.3 centimeters in diameter [80, 81]. The overlying mucosa does not exhibit a change in color or texture. [80]

Pathology and Immunohistochemistry

NSMs have an abundant myxoid matrix and irregular shaped nodules that are bordered with fibrous bands (Figure 13). The cells within the mass are variable in morphology and cytological characteristics. Some cells may be large and multipolar with intracytoplasmic vacuoles of stromal mucin that create a ring appearance. Conversely, small epithelial cells arranged in cords or syncytial aggregates may be observed [2]. Nuclear pleomorphism and mitotic activity are seldom observed [83]. Mast cell are commonly found interspersed within the tissue [82]

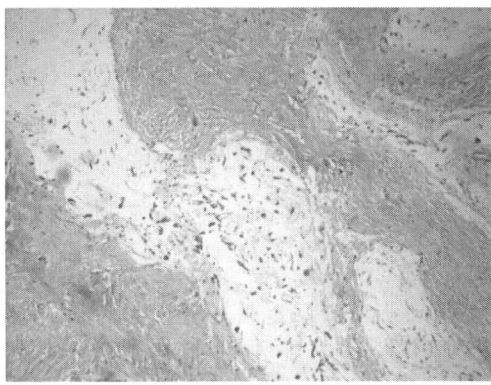

Figure 13. A nerve sheath myxoma characterized by elongated cells loosely arranged against a myxoid matrix. Lobules of the tumor are separated by bands of collagen (hematoxylin and eosin, original magnification 100X).

Immunohistochemically, NSMs stain strongly positive for S-100 protein (Figure 14), vimentin GFAP, neuron specific enolase, and Leu-7. CD34 stains are weakly positive and EMA is variable [80, 83]. Neurothekeomas can be distinguished from true nerve sheath myxomas as they stain positively for NKI/C3 and MiTF but negatively for S-100 and GFAP [2]

The aforementioned features are consistent with the rare oral cases of NSM and no distinct features or patterns were readily appreciated in the review of the literature.

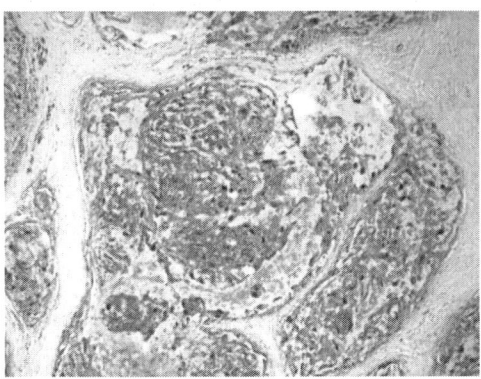

Figure 14. Nerve sheath myxoma demonstrated strong diffuse S-100 immunostaining (original magnification 100X).

Treatment and Outcomes

Treatment, when indicated, consists of wide local excision and recurrence is generally thought to be uncommon, though some studies have found recurrence rates as high as 50% [79, 83]. It is unclear to what extent this relates to incomplete resection. Furthermore, recurrence is rarely documented in NSMs of the oral cavity, though the sample size is inherently small [84]. NSMs are not known to harbor any malignant potential as there are no cases of transformation documented in the literature as of yet.

GRANULAR CELL TUMOR

Etiology

Granular cell tumor (GCT), usually a benign entity, has been referred to in the past by a number of terms such as Abrikossoff's tumor, granular cell myoblastoma, granular cell nerve sheath tumor, and granular cell schwannoma, as our understanding of the tumor etiology has evolved [85,86]. Though it is now universally agreed upon that GCTs have a neurogenic origin, future studies are necessary to unequivocally elucidate the cell of origin. One prominent hypothesis suggests that GCTs derive from undifferentiated mesenchymal cells that that exhibit partial Schwannian differentiation, as this would explain the primarily extraneural topographic distribution of the tumor [87]. They are inconsistently referred to in the literature as any of the following: a true neoplasm, a developmental anomaly, and a reactive proliferative response [21]. Because the incidence of GCT is about twice as high in females (detailed below), a hormonal etiological influence is hypothesized but remains mechanistically uncharacterized and unproven [2]

Epidemiology

GCTs frequently affect the head and neck (45-65% of cases) though they can occur anywhere in the body. Of the head and neck cases, approximately 70% arise intraorally [88]. This tumor class has a particularly high propensity to arise on the tongue and occurs most often in the 4th to 6th decades of life [89]. The next most frequently involved intraoral sites include the buccal mucosa and hard palate [90]. There is some evidence to suggest that females are affected about twice as frequently as males and that persons of black ancestry are affected more frequently, especially in cases of multiple synchronous tumors [91]. Based on a small sample size of 116 patients, malignant GCTs appear to follow many of the same trends as 77% were female, and the median age was 54 years [92]

Clinical Presentation and Diagnosis

Clinically, GCTs usually manifest as a solitary, slow growing, painless nodule that is not easily distinguished from other soft tissue neoplasms [93]. The tumor is described as a well-delimited yellow or pink mass that is less than 3 cm in diameter and covered by an intact overlying mucosa [94, 95]. Pseudoepitheliomatous hyperplasia in the overlying epithelium is a common clinical feature (especially in lesions of the tongue) that can cause the tumor to be confused with squamous cell carcinoma [85]. Some studies document the rate of pseudoepitheliomatous hyperplasia in intraoral GCTs to be upwards of 50% [85, 89, 96]. A superficial biopsy is inadequate as it may only capture the tumor surface hyperplasia while missing other critical distinguishing features [94]. There have been rare but documented cases in which a benign GCT presents with coexisting squamous cell carcinoma at the same site [94]. Pain is atypical in oral lesions, although this has been described [95]. Immunohistochemical evaluation is necessary to differentiate this type of tumor from other entities that exhibit granular cell change. An association has been described between LEOPARD syndrome (mutations in PTPN11) and multiple GCTs [97]

Features indicative of malignancy have been put forth by Fanburg-Smith and requires at least three of the following six criteria: necrosis, tumor cell spindling, vesicular nuclei with large nucleoli, increased rate of mitosis (greater than two mitoses per 10 high-power field), a high nuclear-to-cytoplasmic ratio, and pleomorphism [89, 98, 99]. Tumors that meet one or two of the above criteria are categorized as atypical and their malignant potential is yet to be fully elucidated, though they are thought to be benign [100]. Unfortunately, there are rare examples of tumors without high risk histological features that were confirmed to be metastatic [21]. As such, it is important to always correlate the pathological diagnosis with the clinical presentation.

Pathology and Immunohistochemistry

Granular cell tumors, as the name suggests, invariably demonstrate granular differentiation histologically. Characteristic features of granular differentiation include an abundance of eosinophilic granularity of the cell cytoplasm secondary to the proliferation of lysosomes (Figure 15). Because there are numerous etiologies (and cell types) that can display this histological pattern, such as ameloblastoma, dermatofibroma, oral lichen planus, leiomyoma, angiosarcoma, and melanoma (among others), immunohistochemical staining is critical in order to determine whether or not the cells derive from the neuroectoderm [86]. The cells within the tumor classically exhibit pustule-ovoid bodies of Milian and these appear as round eosinophilic granules that are surrounded by a clear halo. In most cases, the cells appear as polygonal or ovoid in shape with indistinct borders and nuclei that are uniform, hyperchromatic, and peripherally located. Oral lesions specifically have been described with cells arranged in sheets, ribbons, and islands that are separated by fibrous tissue septa [2, 86]. Epidermocytosis is sometimes observed which can cause the lesion to be mistaken as melanoma *in situ* [86]

The immunohistochemical profile for intraoral GCT is characterized by positive periodic acid-Schiff (PAS) staining of cytoplasmic granules and tumor cells that stain positively for S-100 protein, neuron specific enolase, Leu-7, calretinin, vimentin and CD-68 [89, 101]. They do not stain for neurofilament proteins, GFAP, EMA and CD34 [21, 41]. Stains for Ki-67 and p53 can be helpful in differentiating benign from rapidly proliferative malignant lesions [85]. Our understanding of the genetic etiologies and risk factors remains primitive, and although malignant tumors are found to be variously aneuploid, diploid, and hyperdiploid, there is no data to support ploidy as a prognostic marker at this time [86].

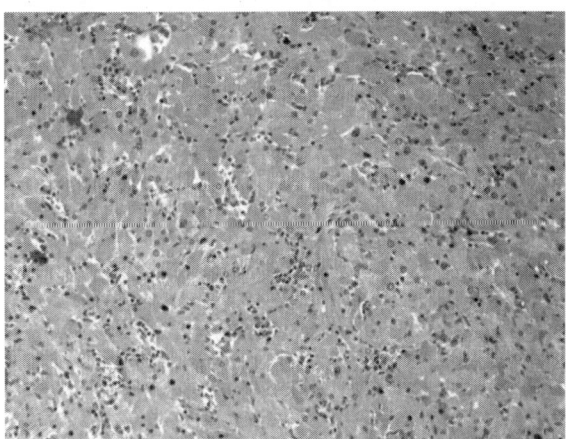

Figure 15. Granular cell tumors are characterized by a granular quality of the tumor cell cytoplasm due to an accumulation of large lysosomes (hematoxylin and eosin, original magnification 200X).

Treatment and Outcomes

Only 1-2% of GCTs are classified as malignant and there is no evidence to suggest that this proportion differs for intraoral GCTs. Definitive surgical resection is the treatment of choice and there is currently no established role for adjuvant chemotherapy or radiation. For lesions that are suspected or proven to be malignant, regional lymph node dissection should be considered, as this is a common site of metastasis [89, 93, 98, 100]. Recurrence of benign lesions is rare but more frequently observed in multifocal disease. Even with incomplete resection, recurrence was only documented in 5 of 24 cases according to one group [102]. Morbidity and mortality are extremely low for benign GCTs [98]. On the other hand, malignant GCTs represent a high-grade sarcoma that has high rates of distant metastasis, recurrence, and poor survival outcomes [99]. The most common sites of metastasis include lymph nodes, bone, liver, and lung [92]

REFERENCES

[1] Perry, Kyle. (2017). "Neural and Nerve Sheath Lesions." In *Soft Tissue Pathology for Clinicians*, edited by Kyle Perry, 123–38. Cham: Springer International Publishing. https://doi.org/10.1007/ 978-3-319-55654-3_9.

[2] Goldblum, John R., Andrew, L. Folpe. & Sharon, W. Weiss. (2014). "Benign Tumors of Peripheral Nerves." In *Enzinger and Weiss's Soft Tissue Tumors*, 6th ed., 784–854. Philadelphia, PA: Elsevier/Saunders. https://www-clinicalkey-com.ccmain.ohionet.org/#!/content/book/3-s2.0-B9780323088343000277.

[3] Michal, Michael., Dmitry, V. Kazakov. & Michal, Michal. (2017). "Hybrid Peripheral Nerve Sheath Tumors: A Review." *Ceskoslovenska Patologie*, *53* (2), 81–88.

[4] Gupta, Tapas K. Das., Richard, D. Brasfield., Elliot, W. Strong. & Steven, I. Hajdu. (1969). "Benign solitary schwannomas (neurilemomas)." *Cancer*, *24* (2), 355–66. https://doi.org/10.1002/1097-0142(196908)24:2<355::AID-CNCR2820240218>3.0.CO;2-2.

[5] Wright, B. A. & Jackson, D. (1980). "Neural Tumors of the Oral Cavity. A Review of the Spectrum of Benign and Malignant Oral Tumors of the Oral Cavity and Jaws." *Oral Surgery, Oral Medicine,*

and *Oral Pathology*, *49* (6), 509–22. https://doi.org/10.1016/0030-4220(80)90075-4.

[6] Salla, Juliana Tito., Aline, Cristina Batista Rodrigues Johann., Bruna, Gonçalves Garcia., Maria, Cássia, Ferreira Aguiar. & Ricardo, Alves Mesquita. (2009). "Retrospective Analysis of Oral Peripheral Nerve Sheath Tumors in Brazilians." *Brazilian Oral Research*, *23* (1), 43–48.

[7] Farid, Mohamad., Elizabeth, G. Demicco., Roberto, Garcia., Linda, Ahn., Pamela, R. Merola., Angela, Cioffi. & Robert, G., Maki. (2014a). "Malignant Peripheral Nerve Sheath Tumors." *The Oncologist*, *19* (2), 193–201. https://doi.org/10.1634/theoncologist.2013-0328.

[8] Wanebo, J. E., Malik, J. M., VandenBerg, S. R., Wanebo, H. J., Driesen, N. & Persing, J. A. (1993). "Malignant Peripheral Nerve Sheath Tumors. A Clinicopathologic Study of 28 Cases." *Cancer*, *71* (4), 1247–53. https://doi.org/10.1002/1097-0142(19930215)71:4<1247::aid-cncr2820710413>3.0.co;2-s.

[9] Kar, Madhabananda., Suryanarayana Deo, S. V., Nootan, Kumar Shukla., Ajay, Malik., Sidharth, DattaGupta., Bidhu, Kumar Mohanti. & Sanjay, Thulkar. (2006). "Malignant Peripheral Nerve Sheath Tumors (MPNST) – Clinicopathological Study and Treatment Outcome of Twenty-Four Cases." *World Journal of Surgical Oncology*, *4* (1), 55. https://doi.org/10.1186/1477-7819-4-55.

[10] Kannan, Ram Abhinav., Kirthi, Koushik., Usha, Muniyappa., Ritika, Harjani. & Arvind, Murthy. (2014). "Malignant Peripheral Nerve Sheath Tumor of Buccal Mucosa: An Oncological Surprise." *American Journal of Medical Case Reports*, *2*, no. 10, 222-224.

[11] Baheti, Akshay D., Ryan, B. O'Malley, Sooah, Kim., Abhishek, R., Keraliya, Sree, Harsha Tirumani., Nikhil, H. Ramaiya. & Carolyn, L. Wang. (2016). "Soft-Tissue Sarcomas: An Update for Radiologists Based on the Revised 2013 World Health Organization Classification." *American Journal of Roentgenology*, *206* (5), 924–32. https://doi.org/10.2214/AJR.15.15498.

[12] Louis, David N., Arie, Perry., Guido, Reifenberger., Andreas, von Deimling., Dominique, Figarella-Branger., Webster, K. Cavenee., Hiroko, Ohgaki., Otmar, D. Wiestler., Paul, Kleihues. & David, W. Ellison. (2016). "The 2016 World Health Organization Classification of Tumors of the Central Nervous System: A Summary." *Acta Neuropathologica*, *131* (6), 803–20. https://doi.org/10.1007/s00401-016-1545-1.

[13] Goldblum, John R., Andrew, L. Folpe. & Sharon, W. Weiss. (2014). "Malignant Peripheral Nerve Sheath Tumors." In *Enzinger and Weiss's Soft Tissue Tumors*, 6th ed., 855–79. Philadelphia, PA: Elsevier/Saunders. https://www-clinicalkey-com.ccmain.ohionet.org/ #!/content/book/3-s2.0-B9780323088343000289?scrollTo=%23hl0000356.

[14] Shintaku, Masayuki., Kyosuke, Wada., Tomoko, Wakasa. & Maho, Ueda. (2011). "Malignant Peripheral Nerve Sheath Tumor with Fibroblastic Differentiation in a Patient with Neurofibromatosis Type 1: Imprint Cytological Findings." *Acta Cytologica*, *55* (5), 467–72. https://doi.org/10.1159/000330676.

[15] Rodriguez, Fausto J., Caterina, Giannini., Robert, J. Spinner. & Arie, Perry. (2018). "Tumors of Peripheral Nerve." In *Practical Surgical Neuropathology: A Diagnostic Approach*, 2nd ed., 323–73. Philadelphia, PA: Elsevier. https://www-clinicalkey-com.ccmain.ohionet.org/#!/content/book/3-s2.0-B9780323449410000151.

[16] Kim, AeRang., Douglas, R. Stewart., Karlyne, M. Reilly., David, Viskochil., Markku, M. Miettinen. & Brigitte, C. Widemann. (2017). "Malignant Peripheral Nerve Sheath Tumors State of the Science: Leveraging Clinical and Biological Insights into Effective Therapies." Research article. Sarcoma, https://doi.org/10.1155/2017/7429697.

[17] Brohl, Andrew S., Elliot, Kahen., Sean, J. Yoder., Jamie, K. Teer. & Damon, R. Reed. (2017). "The Genomic Landscape of Malignant Peripheral Nerve Sheath Tumors: Diverse Drivers of Ras Pathway Activation." *Scientific Reports*, *7* (1), 1–5. https://doi.org/10.1038/s41598-017-15183-1.

[18] Korfhage, Justin. & David, B. Lombard. (2019). "Malignant Peripheral Nerve Sheath Tumors: From Epigenome to Bedside." *Molecular Cancer Research: MCR*, *17* (7), 1417–28. https://doi.org/10.1158/1541-7786.MCR-19-0147.

[19] Öztürk, Özmen. & Alper, Tutkun. (2012). "A Case Report of a Malignant Peripheral Nerve Sheath Tumor of the Oral Cavity in Neurofibromatosis Type 1." *Case Reports in Otolaryngology*, https://doi.org/10.1155/2012/936735.

[20] Goldblum, John R., Andrew, L. Folpe. & Sharon, W. Weiss. (2014). "Malignant Peripheral Nerve Sheath Tumors." In *Enzinger and Weiss's Soft Tissue Tumors*, 6th ed., 855–79. Philadelphia, PA: Elsevier/Saunders. https://www-clinicalkey-com.ccmain.ohionet.org/ #!/content/book/3-s2.0-B9780323088343000289?scrollTo=%23hl0000356.

[21] Bouquot, Jerry E., Susan, Muller. & Hiromasa, Nikai. (2009). "Lesions of the Oral Cavity." In *Diagnostic Surgical Pathology of the Head and Neck*, 2nd ed., 191–308. Philadelphia, PA: Elsevier/Saunders. https://www-clinicalkey-com.ccmain.ohionet.org/#!/content/book/3 s2.0 B9781416025894000048?scrollTo=%23hl0003979.

[22] Ng, Vincent Y., Thomas, J. Scharschmidt, Joel, L. Mayerson. & James, L. Fisher. (2013). "Incidence and Survival in Sarcoma in the United States: A Focus on Musculoskeletal Lesions." *Anticancer Research*, *33* (6), 2597–2604.

[23] Roy, Soumyajit., Ajeet, Kumar Gandhi., Bharti, Devnani., Lavleen, Singh. & Bidhu, Kalyan Mohanti. (2017). "Malignant Peripheral Nerve Sheath Tumor of the Tongue with an Unusual Pattern of Recurrence." *Journal of the Egyptian National Cancer Institute*, *29* (2), 115–18. https://doi.org/10.1016/j.jnci.2016.11.001.

[24] Minovi, Amir., Oliver, Basten., Ben, Hunter., Wolfgang, Draf. & Ulrike, Bockmühl. (2007). "Malignant peripheral nerve sheath tumors of the head and neck: Management of 10 cases and literature review." *Head & Neck*, *29* (5), 439–45. https://doi.org/10.1002/hed.20537.

[25] Stark, A. M., Buhl, R., Hugo, H. H. & Mehdorn, H. M. (2001). "Malignant Peripheral Nerve Sheath Tumours – Report of 8 Cases and Review of the Literature." *Acta Neurochirurgica*, *143* (4), 357–64. https://doi.org/10.1007/s007010170090.

[26] Maharudrappa, B. & Kumar, G. S. (2011). "Neural Tumours of Oral and Para Oral Region." *International Journal of Dental Clinics*, *3* (1), http://www.intjdc.com/index.php/intjdc/article/view/236.

[27] Kumar, Priya., Varun, Surya., Aadithya, B. Urs., Augustine, J., Sujata, Mohanty. & Sunita, Gupta. (2019). "Sarcomas of the Oral and Maxillofacial Region: Analysis of 26 Cases with Emphasis on Diagnostic Challenges." *Pathology Oncology Research: POR*, *25* (2), 593–601. https://doi.org/10.1007/s12253-018-0510-9.

[28] Wei, Shi., Evita, Henderson-Jackson., Xiaohua, Qian. & Marilyn, M. Bui. (2017). "Soft Tissue Tumor Immunohistochemistry Update: Illustrative Examples of Diagnostic Pearls to Avoid Pitfalls." *Archives of Pathology & Laboratory Medicine*, *141* (8), 1072–91. https://doi.org/10.5858/arpa.2016-0417-RA.

[29] Hirose, Takanori., Takayuki, Tani., Tetsuya, Shimada., Keisuke, Ishizawa., Shio, Shimada. & Toshiaki, Sano. (2003). "Immunohistochemical Demonstration of EMA/Glut1-Positive Perineurial Cells and CD34-Positive Fibroblastic Cells in Peripheral Nerve Sheath Tumors." *Modern Pathology*, *16* (4), 293–98. https://doi.org/10.1097/01.MP.0000062654.83617.B7.

[30] Janardhanan, Mahija., Rakesh, S. & Vinod Kumar, R. B. (2011). "Intraoral Presentation of Multiple Malignant Peripheral Nerve Sheath Tumors Associated with Neurofibromatosis-1." *Journal of Oral and Maxillofacial Pathology: JOMFP*, *15* (1), 46–51. https://doi.org/10.4103/0973-029X.80025.

[31] Karajannis, Matthias A. & Anat, Stemmer-Rachamimov. (2015). "Schwannomas." In *Molecular Pathology of Nervous System Tumors: Biological Stratification and Targeted Therapies*, edited by Matthias A. Karajannis and David Zagzag, 201–11. Molecular Pathology Library. New York, NY: Springer New York. https://doi.org/10.1007/978-1-4939-1830-0_15.

[32] Hatziotia, J. C. & Asprides, H. (1967). "Neurilemoma (Schwannoma) or the Oral Cavity." *Oral Surgery, Oral Medicine, and Oral Pathology*, 24 (4), 510–26. https://doi.org/10.1016/0030-4220(67)90431-8.

[33] Metwaly, Hamdy., Satoshi, Maruyama., Jun, Cheng., Hideyuki, Hoshina., Ritsuo, Takagi., Takafumi, Hayashi. & Takashi, Saku. (2010). "Central Schwannoma of the Mandible: Report of a Case and Review of the Literature." *Oral Medicine & Pathology*, 15 (1), 29–33. https://doi.org/10.3353/omp.15.29.

[34] Chi, Angela C., John, Carey. & Susan, Muller. (2003). "Intraosseous Schwannoma of the Mandible: A Case Report and Review of the Literature." *Oral Surgery, Oral Medicine, Oral Pathology, Oral Radiology, and Endodontology*, 96 (1), 54–65. https://doi.org/10.1016/ S1079-2104(03)00228-2.

[35] George, N. A., Wagh, M., Balagopal, P. G., Gupta, S., Sukumaran, R. & Sebastian, P. (2014). "Schwannoma Base Tongue: Case Report and Review of Literature." *The Gulf Journal of Oncology*, 1 (16), 94–100.

[36] Kurup, Seema., Krishnakumar, Thankappan., Nitin, Krishnan. & Preeti, P. Nair. (2012). "Intraoral Schwannoma – a Report of Two Cases." *Case Reports*, (July), bcr1220115389. https://doi.org/10.1136/bcr.12.2011.5389.

[37] De Luca-Johnson, Javier. & Alexandra, N. Kalof. (2016). "Peripheral Nerve Sheath Tumors: An Update and Review of Diagnostic Challenges." *Diagnostic Histopathology, Mini-Symposium: Neuropathology*, 22 (11), 447–57. https://doi.org/10.1016/j.mpdhp.2016.10.008.

[38] Santos, Pedro Paulo de Andrade., Valéria, Souza Freitas., Leão, Pereira Pinto., Roseana, de Almeida Freitas. & Lélia, Batista de Souza. (2010). "Clinicopathologic Analysis of 7 Cases of Oral Schwannoma and Review of the Literature." *Annals of Diagnostic Pathology*, 14 (4), 235–39. https://doi.org/10.1016/ j.anndiagpath.2010.02.009.

[39] Thompson, Lester D. R., Stephen, S. Koh. & Sean, K. Lau. (2019). "Tongue Schwannoma: A Clinicopathologic Study of 19 Cases."

Head and Neck Pathology, September. https://doi.org/10.1007/s12105-019-01071-9.

[40] Muruganandhan, J., Srinivasa Prasad, T., Selvakumar, T. & Nalin, Kumar S. (2013). "Ancient Neurilemmoma: A Rare Oral Tumor." *Journal of Oral and Maxillofacial Pathology : JOMFP*, *17* (3), 447–50. https://doi.org/10.4103/0973-029X.125218.

[41] Campos, Marcia Sampaio., Alexandra, Fontes., Luciana, Sassa Marocchio., Fabio, Daumas Nunes. & Suzana, Cantanhede Orsini Machado de Sousa. (2012). "Clinicopathologic and Immunohistochemical Features of Oral Neurofibroma." *Acta Odontologica Scandinavica*, *70* (6), 577–82. https://doi.org/10.3109/00016357.2011.640286.

[42] Yang, Shih-Wei. & Chin-Yew, Lin. (2003). "Schwannoma of the Upper Lip: Case Report and Literature Review." *American Journal of Otolaryngology*, *24* (5), 351–54. https://doi.org/10.1016/s0196-0709(03)00065-6.

[43] Lee, Edwin J., Thomas, C. Calcaterra. & Lionel, Zuckerbraun. (1998). "Traumatic Neuromas of the Head and Neck." *Ear, Nose & Throat Journal;* New York, *77* (8), 670–74, 676.

[44] Eguchi, Takanori., Rikuma, Ishida., Hironori, Ara., Yoshiki, Hamada, & Ikuyo, Kanai. (2016). "A Diffuse Traumatic Neuroma in the Palate: A Case Report." *Journal of Medical Case Reports*, *10* (1), 116. https://doi.org/10.1186/s13256-016-0908-5.

[45] Oliveira, Karla M. C., Lukas, Pindur., Zhihua, Han., Mit, B. Bhavsar., John, H. Barker. & Liudmila, Leppik. (2018). "Time Course of Traumatic Neuroma Development." *PLoS ONE*, *13* (7). https://doi.org/10.1371/journal.pone.0200548.

[46] Jones, A. V. & Franklin, C. D. (2006). "An Analysis of Oral and Maxillofacial Pathology Found in Adults over a 30-Year Period." *Journal of Oral Pathology & Medicine: Official Publication of the International Association of Oral Pathologists and the American Academy of Oral Pathology*, *35* (7), 392–401. https://doi.org/10.1111/j.1600-0714.2006.00451.x.

[47] Sist, Thomas C. & George, W. Greene. (1981). "Traumatic Neuroma of the Oral Cavity: Report of Thirty-One New Cases and Review of the Literature." *Oral Surgery, Oral Medicine, Oral Pathology, 51* (4), 394–402. https://doi.org/10.1016/0030-4220(81)90149-3.

[48] Murphey, M. D., Smith, W. S., Smith, S. E., Kransdorf, M. J. & Temple, H. T. (1999). "From the Archives of the AFIP. Imaging of Musculoskeletal Neurogenic Tumors: Radiologic-Pathologic Correlation." *Radiographics: A Review Publication of the Radiological Society of North America, Inc, 19* (5), 1253–80. https://doi.org/10.1148/radiographics.19.5.g99se101253.

[49] Suramya, S., Pratibha, Shashikumar., Shreeshyla, H. S. & Sheela, Kumar G. (2013). "Solitary Plexiform Neurofibroma of the Gingiva: Unique Presentation in the Oral Cavity." *Journal of Clinical and Diagnostic Research: JCDR, 7* (9), 2090–92. https://doi.org/10.7860/JCDR/2013/6535.3416.

[50] Venkataswamy, Asha Reddy., Shesha, Prasad Ranganath., Sri, Manasa Challapalli. & Leeky, Mohanthy. (2016). "Nonsyndromic solitary neurofibromas in the oral cavity: Case series and literature review." *Journal of Indian Academy of Oral Medicine and Radiology, 28*, no. 1, 52.

[51] Mahalle, Aditi., Mamatha, G. S. Reddy., Supriya, Mohit Kheur., Neta, Bagul. & Yashwant, Ingle. (2016). "Solitary Non Syndromic Oral Plexiform Neurofibroma: A Case Report and Review of Literature." *Journal of Dentistry, 17*, (3 Suppl), 293–96.

[52] Jouhilahti, Eeva-Mari., Sirkku, Peltonen., Anthony, M. Heape. & Juha, Peltonen. (2011). "The Pathoetiology of Neurofibromatosis 1." *The American Journal of Pathology, 178* (5), 1932–39. https://doi.org/ 10.1016/j.ajpath.2010.12.056.

[53] Al-Omran, Mohammed K., Abdul-Nabi, K. Al-Khamis. & Ashok, K. Malik. (2006). "Solitary Neurofibroma of the Floor of the Mouth." *Neurosciences (Riyadh, Saudi Arabia), 11* (1), 53–55.

[54] Geist, J. R., Gander, D. L. & Stefanac, S. J. (1992). "Oral Manifestations of Neurofibromatosis Types I and II." *Oral Surgery, Oral Medicine, and Oral Pathology, 73* (3), 376–82.

[55] Messersmith, Lynn. & Kevin, Krauland. (2019). "Neurofibroma." In *StatPearls [Internet]*. StatPearls Publishing, http://www.ncbi.nlm.nih.gov/books/NBK539707/.

[56] Jangam, Sagar Satish., Snehal, Nilesh Ingole., Mohan, Devidas Deshpande. & Pallavi, Adinath Ranadive. (2014). "Solitary Intraosseous Neurofibroma: Report of a Unique Case." *Contemporary Clinical Dentistry*, 5 (4), 561–63. https://doi.org/10.4103/0976-237X.142833.

[57] Mahmud, Sk. Abdul., Neha, Shah., Moumita, Chattaraj. & Swagata, Gayen. (2016). "Solitary Encapsulated Neurofibroma Not Associated with Neurofibromatosis-1 Affecting Tongue in a 73-Year-Old Female." *Case Reports in Dentistry*, https://doi.org/10.1155/2016/3630153.

[58] Friedman, J. M. & Birch, P. H. (1997). "Type 1 Neurofibromatosis: A Descriptive Analysis of the Disorder in 1,728 Patients." *American Journal of Medical Genetics*, 70 (2), 138–43.

[59] Gómez-Oliveira, Guillermo., Javier, Fernández-Alba Luengo., Roberto, Martín-Sastre., Beatriz, Patiño-Seijas. & José, Luis López-Cedrún-Cembranos. (2004). "Plexiform Neurofibroma of the Cheek Mucosa. A Case Report." *Medicina Oral: Organo Oficial De La Sociedad Espanola De Medicina Oral Y De La Academia Iberoamericana De Patologia Y Medicina Bucal*, 9 (3), 263–67.

[60] Neville, B. W., Hann, J., Narang, R. & Garen, P. (1991). "Oral Neurofibrosarcoma Associated with Neurofibromatosis Type I." *Oral Surgery, Oral Medicine, and Oral Pathology*, 72 (4), 456–61. https://doi.org/10.1016/0030-4220(91)90560-y.

[61] Koutlas, Ioannis G. & Bernd, W. Scheithauer. (2010). "Palisaded Encapsulated ('Solitary Circumscribed') Neuroma of the Oral Cavity: A Review of 55 Cases." *Head and Neck Pathology*, 4 (1), 15–26. https://doi.org/10.1007/s12105-010-0162-x.

[62] Mortazavi, Nazanin., Azadeh, Gholami., Pouyan, Amini Shakib. & Hamed, Hosseinkazemi. (2015). "Palisaded Encapsulated Neuroma of the Tongue Clinically Mimicking a Pyogenic Granuloma: A Case

Report and Review of Literature." *Journal of Dentistry (Tehran, Iran)*, *12* (7), 537–41.
[63] Magnusson, B. (1996). "Palisaded Encapsulated Neuroma (Solitary Circumscribed Neuroma) of the Oral Mucosa." *Oral Surgery, Oral Medicine, Oral Pathology, Oral Radiology, and Endodontics*, *82* (3), 302–4. https://doi.org/10.1016/s1079-2104(96)80356-8.
[64] Atarbashi-Moghadam, Saede., Ali, Lotfi., Saman, Salehi Zalani. & Sepideh, Mokhtari. (2017). "Palisaded Encapsulated (Solitary Circumscribed) Neuroma of the Buccal Mucosa: A Rare Case." *Journal of Dentistry*, *18* (4), 314–17.
[65] Batra, Jaskaran., Ramesh, V., Anupama, Molpariya. & Khushpreet, K. Maan. (2018). "Palisaded Encapsulated Neuroma: An Unusual Presentation." *Indian Dermatology Online Journal*, *9* (4), 262–64. https://doi.org/10.4103/idoj.IDOJ_354_17.
[66] Manchanda, Adesh S., Ramandeep, Singh Narang. & Geetika, Puri. (2015). "Palisaded Encapsulated Neuroma." *Journal of Orofacial Sciences*, *7* (2), 136. https://doi.org/10.4103/0975-8844.164308.
[67] Rodriguez, Fausto J., Andrew, L. Folpe., Caterina, Giannini. & Arie, Perry. (2012). "Pathology of Peripheral Nerve Sheath Tumors: Diagnostic Overview and Update on Selected Diagnostic Problems." *Acta Neuropathologica*, *123* (3), 295–319. https://doi.org/10.1007/s00401-012-0954-z.
[68] Mariño-Enríquez, Adrián. & Jason, L. Hornick. (2019). "Spindle Cell Tumors of Adults." In *Practical Soft Tissue Pathology: A Diagnostic Approach*, 2nd ed., 15–100. Philadelphia, PA: Elsevier. https://www-clinicalkey-com.ccmain.ohionet.org/#!/content/book/3-s2.0-B978032349714500003X.
[69] Rocha, Lília Alves., Sílvia, Maria Paparotto Lopes., Alan, Roger dos Santos Silva., Márcio, Ajudarte Lopes. & Pablo, Agustin Vargas. (2009). "Oral Intraneural Perineurioma: Report of Two Cases." *Clinics*, *64* (10), 1037–39. https://doi.org/10.1590/S1807-59322009001000017.
[70] Schadel, Caleb M., Craig, W. Anderson., Angela, C. Chi. & Martin, B. Steed. (2019). "Perineurioma of the Tongue: A Case Report and

Review of the Literature." *Journal of Oral and Maxillofacial Surgery: Official Journal of the American Association of Oral and Maxillofacial Surgeons*, 77 (2), 329.e1-329.e7. https://doi.org/10.1016/j.joms.2018.09.032.

[71] Macarenco, Ricardo S., Fred, Ellinger. & Andre, M. Oliveira. (2007). "Perineurioma: A Distinctive and Underrecognized Peripheral Nerve Sheath Neoplasm." *Archives of Pathology & Laboratory Medicine*, 131 (4), 625–36. https://doi.org/10.1043/1543-2165(2007)131[625: PADAUP]2.0.CO;2.

[72] Huang, Yong., Hongwei, Li., Zhengwen, Xiong. & Rui, Chen. (2014). "Intraneural Malignant Perineurioma: A Case Report and Review of Literature." *International Journal of Clinical and Experimental Pathology*, 7 (7), 4503–7.

[73] Gordon, Catherine M., Joseph, A. Majzoub., Debbie, J. Marsh., John, B. Mulliken., Bruce, A. J. Ponder., Bruce, G. Robinson. & Charis, Eng. (1998). "Four Cases of Mucosal Neuroma Syndrome: Multiple Endocrine Neoplasm 2B or Not 2B?" *The Journal of Clinical Endocrinology & Metabolism*, 83 (1), 17–20. https://doi.org/10.1210/jcem.83.1.4504.

[74] Lima, Rubianne Ligório de. (2016). "Rare Mucosal Neuroma on the Basis of Language: Case Report." *Global Journal of Otolaryngology*, 2 (5). https://doi.org/10.19080/GJO.2016.02.555596.

[75] Shimazaki, Takatsugu., Yoshikazu, Yoshida., Shinsuke, Izumaru. & Tadashi, Nakashima. (2003). "Laryngeal Solitary Multiple Mucosal Neuromas without Multiple Endocrine Neoplasia (MEN) Type 2B." *Auris Nasus Larynx*, 30 (2), 191–95. https://doi.org/10.1016/S0385-8146(02)00115-3.

[76] Nishihara, Kazunari., Hiroshi, Yoshida., Kojiro, Onizawa., Hiroshi, Yusa. & Masachika, Fujiwara. (2004). "Solitary Mucosal Neuroma of the Hard Palate: A Case Report." *The British Journal of Oral & Maxillofacial Surgery*, 42 (5), 457–59. https://doi.org/10.1016/j.bjoms.2004.04.007.

[77] Znaczko, Anna., Deirdre, E. Donnelly. & Patrick, J. Morrison. (2014). "Epidemiology, Clinical Features, and Genetics of Multiple

Endocrine Neoplasia Type 2B in a Complete Population." *The Oncologist*, *19* (12), 1284–86. https://doi.org/10.1634/ theoncologist. 2014-0277.

[78] Lee, Min Jung., Ki, Hun Chung., Joon, Soo Park., Hyun, Chung., Hyo, Chan Jang. & Jong, Won Kim. (2010). "Multiple Endocrine Neoplasia Type 2B: Early Diagnosis by Multiple Mucosal Neuroma and Its DNA Analysis." *Annals of Dermatology*, *22* (4), 452–55. https://doi.org/10. 5021/ad.2010.22.4.452.

[79] Rozza-de-Menezes, Rafaela Elvira., Raquel, Machado Andrade., Mônica, Simões Israel. & Karin, Soares Gonçalves Cunha. (2013). "Intraoral Nerve Sheath Myxoma: Case Report and Systematic Review of the Literature." *Head & Neck*, *35* (12), E397–404. https://doi.org/10.1002/hed.23361.

[80] Nishioka, Mai., Rodelio, L. Aguirre., Ayataka, Ishikawa., Kiyoko, Nagumo., Li-Hong, Wang. & Norihiko, Okada. (2009). "Nerve Sheath Myxoma (Neurothekeoma) Arising in the Oral Cavity: Histological and Immunohistochemical Features of 3 Cases." *Oral Surgery, Oral Medicine, Oral Pathology, Oral Radiology, and Endodontology*, *107* (5), e28–33. https://doi.org/10.1016/j.tripleo. 2009.01.018.

[81] Safadi, Rima A., John, W. Hellstein., May, M. Diab. & Huda, M. Hammad. (2010). "Nerve Sheath Myxoma (Neurothekeoma) of the Gingiva, A Case Report and Review of the Literature." *Head and Neck Pathology*, *4* (3), 242–45. https://doi.org/10.1007/s12105-010-0183-5.

[82] Frydrych, Agnieszka M. & Norman, A. Firth. (2017). "Oral Nerve Sheath Myxoma: A Rare and Unusual Intraoral Neoplasm." *Clinical Case Reports*, *6* (2), 302–5. https://doi.org/ 10.1002/ccr3.1341.

[83] Bhat, Amoolya., Aparna, Narasimha., Vijaya, C. & Sundeep, V. K. (2015). "Nerve Sheath Myxoma: Report of A Rare Case." *Journal of Clinical and Diagnostic Research : JCDR*, *9* (4), ED07–9. https://doi. org/10.7860/JCDR/2015/10911.5810.

[84] Tiffee, John C. & Donald, R. Pulitzer. (1996). "Nerve Sheath Myxoma of the Oral Cavity." *Oral Surgery, Oral Medicine, Oral Pathology, Oral Radiology, and Endodontology, 82* (4), 423–25. https://doi.org/10.1016/S1079-2104(96)80308-8.

[85] Eguia, Asier., Agurne, Uribarri., Cosme, Gay Escoda., Miguel, Angel Crovetto., Rafael, Martínez-Conde. & Jose, Manuel Aguirre. (2006). "Granular Cell Tumor: Report of 8 Intraoral Cases." *Medicina Oral, Patologia Oral Y Cirugia Bucal, 11* (5), E425-428.

[86] Cardis, Michael A., Jonathan, Ni. & Jag, Bhawan. (2017). "Granular Cell Differentiation: A Review of the Published Work." *The Journal of Dermatology, 44* (3), 251–58. https://doi.org/10.1111/1346-8138.13758.

[87] Chow, Louis T. C. & Maria, B. C. Y. Chow. (2019). "Intraneural Granular Cell Tumor: Histologic Spectrum and Histogenetic Implication." *Journal of Cutaneous Pathology*, August. https://doi.org/10.1111/cup.13558.

[88] Dive, Alka., Akshay, Dhobley., Prajakta, Zade Fande. & Sudhanshu, Dixit. (2013). "Granular Cell Tumor of the Tongue: Report of a Case." *Journal of Oral and Maxillofacial Pathology : JOMFP, 17* (1), 148. https://doi.org/10.4103/0973-029X.110728.

[89] Loo, Sander van de., Erik, Thunnissen., Pieter, Postmus. & Isaäc, van der Waal. (2015). "Granular Cell Tumor of the Oral Cavity; a Case Series Including a Case of Metachronous Occurrence in the Tongue and the Lung." *Medicina Oral, Patología Oral y Cirugía Bucal, 20* (1), e30–33. https://doi.org/10.4317/medoral.19867.

[90] Nagaraj, Praveen Birur., Ravikiran, Ongole. & Balaji, Rao Bhujanga Rao. (2006). "Granular Cell Tumor of the Tongue in a 6-Year-Old Girl: A Case Report." *Medicina Oral, Patología Oral y Cirugía Bucal (Internet), 11* (2), 162–64.

[91] Goodstein, M. L., Eisele, D. W., Hyams, V. J. & Kashima, H. K. (1990). "Multiple Synchronous Granular Cell Tumors of the Upper Aerodigestive Tract." *Otolaryngology--Head and Neck Surgery: Official Journal of American Academy of Otolaryngology-Head*

and Neck Surgery, 103 (4), 664–68. https://doi.org/10.1177/019459989010300426.

[92] Moten, Ambria S., Huaqing, Zhao., Hong, Wu. & Jeffrey, M. Farma. (2018). "Malignant Granular Cell Tumor: Clinical Features and Long-Term Survival." *Journal of Surgical Oncology*, 118 (6), 891–97. https://doi.org/10.1002/jso.25227.

[93] Cui, Ying., Shan-Shan, Tong., Yan-Hong, Zhang. & Hui-Ting, Li. (2018). "Granular Cell Tumor: A Report of Three Cases and Review of Literature." *Cancer Biomarkers: Section A of Disease Markers*, 23 (2), 173–78. https://doi.org/10.3233/CBM-170556.

[94] Sena, Costa., Nivea, Cristina., Fernanda, Bertini., Yasmin, Rodarte Carvalho., Janete, Dias Almeida. & Ana, Sueli Rodrigues Cavalcante. (2012). "Granular Cell Tumor Presenting as a Tongue Nodule: Two Case Reports." *Journal of Medical Case Reports*, 6 (1), 56. https://doi.org/10.1186/1752-1947-6-56.

[95] Collins, B. M. & Jones, A. C. (1995). "Multiple Granular Cell Tumors of the Oral Cavity: Report of a Case and Review of the Literature." *Journal of Oral and Maxillofacial Surgery: Official Journal of the American Association of Oral and Maxillofacial Surgeons*, 53 (6), 707–11. https://doi.org/10.1016/0278-2391(95)90178-7.

[96] Ferreira, Jean Carlos Barbosa., Angélica, Ferreira Oton-Leite., Rafaela, Guidi. & Elismauro, Francisco Mendonça. (2017). "Granular Cell Tumor Mimicking a Squamous Cell Carcinoma of the Tongue: A Case Report." *BMC Research Notes*, 10, (January). https://doi.org/10.1186/s13104-016-2325-7.

[97] Schrader, K. A., Nelson, T. N., De Luca, A., Huntsman, D. G. & McGillivray, B. C. (2009). "Multiple Granular Cell Tumors Are an Associated Feature of LEOPARD Syndrome Caused by Mutation in PTPN11." *Clinical Genetics*, 75 (2), 185–89. https://doi.org/10.1111/j.1399-0004.2008.01100.x.

[98] Moten, Ambria S., Sujana, Movva., Margaret, von Mehren., Hong, Wu., Nestor, F. Esnaola., Sanjay, S. Reddy. & Jeffrey, M. Farma. (2018). "Granular Cell Tumor Experience at a Comprehensive Cancer

Center." *The Journal of Surgical Research*, *226*, 1–7. https://doi.org/10.1016/j.jss.2018.01.027.

[99] Fanburg-Smith, J. C., Meis-Kindblom, J. M., Fante, R. & Kindblom, L. G. (1998). "Malignant Granular Cell Tumor of Soft Tissue: Diagnostic Criteria and Clinicopathologic Correlation." *The American Journal of Surgical Pathology*, *22* (7), 779–94. https://doi.org/10.1097/00000478-199807000-00001.

[100] Alnashwan, Yara A., Khaled, A. H. Ali. & Samir, S. Amr. (2019). "Metastasizing Malignant Granular Cell Tumor (Abrikossoff Tumor) of the Anterior Abdominal Wall, with Prolonged Survival." Research article. *Case Reports in Pathology.*, 2019. https://doi.org/10.1155/2019/9576487.

[101] Chrysomali, Evanthia., Stavros, I Papanicolaou., Nusi, P Dekker. & Joseph, A Regezi. (1997). "Benign Neural Tumors of the Oral Cavity: A Comparative Immunohistochemical Study." *Oral Surgery, Oral Medicine, Oral Pathology, Oral Radiology, and Endodontology* 84 (4): 381–90. https://doi.org/10.1016/S1079-2104(97)90036-6.

[102] Lack, E. E., Worsham, G. F., Callihan, M. D., Crawford, B. E., Klappenbach, S., Rowden, G. & Chun, B. (1980). "Granular Cell Tumor: A Clinicopathologic Study of 110 Patients." *Journal of Surgical Oncology*, *13* (4), 301–16. https://doi.org/10.1002/jso.2930130405.

In: Nerve Sheath Tumors
Editor: Richard A. Prayson

ISBN: 978-1-53617-366-6
© 2020 Nova Science Publishers, Inc.

Chapter 4

CLINICOPATHOLOGIC FEATURES OF SALIVARY GLAND PERIPHERAL NERVE SHEATH TUMORS

Brigid E. Prayson, BA and *Richard A. Prayson*[*], *MD, MEd*

The Ohio State University College of Medicine and Cleveland Clinic Department of Anatomic Pathology

ABSTRACT

Salivary gland peripheral nerve sheath tumors are relatively rare neoplasms and their diagnosis is usually not expected preoperatively. Most of the literature focused on the three main tumors in this grouping (schwannomas, neurofibromas, and malignant peripheral nerve sheath tumors) consists of case reports and small series. An association of neurofibromas and plexiform neurofibromas with Neurofibromatosis type I is well documented. The benign tumors (schwannomas and neurofibromas) typically present as slow growing, painless, mobile masses. Malignant peripheral nerve sheath tumors may be painful or non

---

[*] Corresponding Author's Email: praysor@ccf.org; Fax: 216-445-6967.

painful masses that often are associated with sudden increased growth. The tumors morphologically resemble their counterparts in other regions of the body. This chapter will review the literature on these three tumor types arising in salivary gland tissue and summarize the clinicopathologic features of these neoplasms.

Keywords: salivary glands, salivary gland tumors, schwannoma, neurofibroma, malignant peripheral nerve sheath tumor

INTRODUCTION

The three paired salivary glands include the parotid, submandibular and sublingual glands. Each is associated with peripheral nerve tissue. The facial nerve, great auricular nerve and auriculotemporal nerves are situated in and adjacent to the parotid glands. The submandibular glands are associated with the facial nerves (marginal mandibular branches), lingual nerves and hypoglossal nerves. The sublingual glands are the smallest of the paired salivary glands and are associated with the chorda tympani and the lingual branch of the mandibular nerve. On rare occasion, peripheral nerve sheath tumors may arise from one of the aforementioned nerves and present as a salivary gland based mass. This chapter will focus on the three most common peripheral nerve sheath tumors to arise in this setting (neurofibromas, schwannomas and malignant peripheral nerve sheath tumors).

In 2008, Kyung-Ja Cho and colleagues reviewed the surgical pathology files of the Asian Medical Center during a 7 year period to identify intraparenchymal mesenchymal tumors of the salivary glands [1]. Of the 18 cases of intraparenchymal mesenchymal salivary gland tumors they identified, six were schwannomas and one was a plexiform neurofibroma. More recently, Guraya and Prayson found only nine patients with peripheral nerve sheath tumors arising in the salivary glands over a 25 year period in their institutional review, including five neurofibromas, three schwannomas and one malignant peripheral nerve sheath tumor [2].

NEUROFIBROMAS

A neurofibroma may present with a variety of growth pattern types including a diffuse growth pattern, localized intraneural pattern, and a plexiform growth pattern. They may arise as isolated lesions or in association with other neurofibromas in the setting of Neurofibromatosis type I, an autosomal dominant, genetically inherited disease caused by a germline mutation in the NF1 tumor suppressor gene located on chromosome 17q11.2 which encodes for neurofibromin. Neurofibromas can arise at any age, and when they arise in the salivary glands, they have been most commonly encountered in the parotid gland, although rare tumors have been reported to originate in the submandibular gland [2-5]. Salivary gland tumors appear to show a male predilection [2, 3]. Patients most commonly present with a unilateral, nontender and often mobile mass; the overlying skin is typically spared [3, 6-8]. Patients with facial nerve tumors may present with symptoms related to nerve compression such as facial droop but usually do not present with symptoms secondary to dysfunction of the nerve itself, such as pain or paresthesias [2, 6, 9, 10]. Imaging studies usually show a mass that resembles a benign tumor which can not be reliably distinguished from other benign masses of the salivary gland. Magnetic resonance imaging (MRI) studies may show a well demarcated, slightly heterogenously enhancing mass [10, 11].

Microscopically, neurofibromas are marked by elongated Schwann cells arranged in wavy bundles against a loose, mucoid type background (Figure 1). Occasional mast cells are sprinkled throughout the tumor. The cells demonstrate little in the way of nuclear pleomorphism (Figure 1). Mitotic figures are only rarely seen. In longstanding tumors, increased collagen deposition may be present. Occasional tumors may be marked by focal areas of increased cellularity (cellular neurofibroma) but little cytologic atypia or mitotic activity. Other tumors may show some degree of degenerative nuclear atypia (atypical neurofibroma) with little or no proliferative activity. These variants are important to distinguish from malignant peripheral nerve sheath tumors, which arise from neurofibromas. The tumor may be circumscribed or locally infiltrate adjacent structures (Figure 2). A subset of tumors grow in a plexiform pattern, characterized by multiple fascicles that have been likened to a "bag of worms" (Figure 3). The plexiform variant is particularly associated with Neurofibromatosis type I and is more likely to undergo malignant degeneration over time.

Neurofibromas, being primarily Schwann cell derived, generally stain with antibodies to S-100 protein and SOX 10. The fibroblastic component of the neurofibroma can be highlighted with vimentin antibody. Perineurial cells, which are present in smaller numbers, can be highlighted with epithelial membrane antigen (EMA) antibody. Neurofilament staining may highlight overrun or entrapped axons in the tumor. Ultrastructural findings mirror the heterogenous cellular composition of the tumor [12].

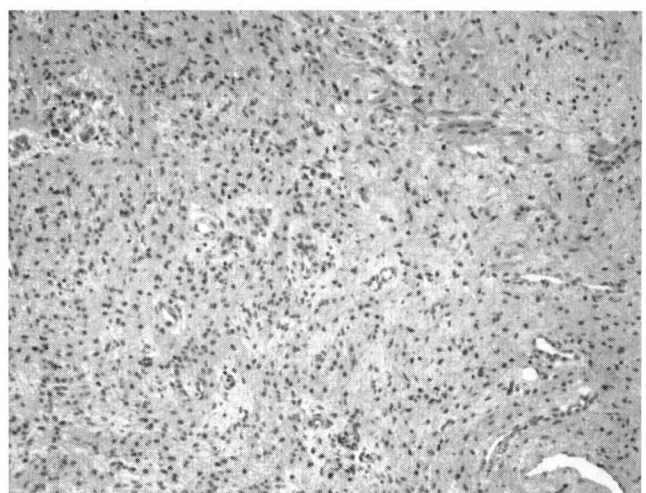

Figure 1. Neurofibroma of the parotid gland marked by cells with an elongated appearance arranged against a loose background. Minimal nuclear pleomorphism is seen (hematoxylin and eosin, original magnification 200X).

Because of the intraoperative risk of damaging the facial nerve or compromising its function, along with the benign nature of the tumor, radical resection of neurofibromas is generally not recommended [2]. Overall, surgical excision is the treatment of choice. With neurofibromas, nerve fibers tend to be incorporated in the tumor and resection of the tumor also means resection of accompanying intermixed nerve tissue [10]. Follow up of patients long term is recommended, particularly in the setting of tumors arising in Neurofibromatosis type I for two reasons. New tumors may arise in the setting of Neurofibromatosis type I and a subset of neurofibromas, 10-15%, may undergo malignant transformation [9, 14]. Tumors that become malignant often present with pain and sudden tumor enlargement.

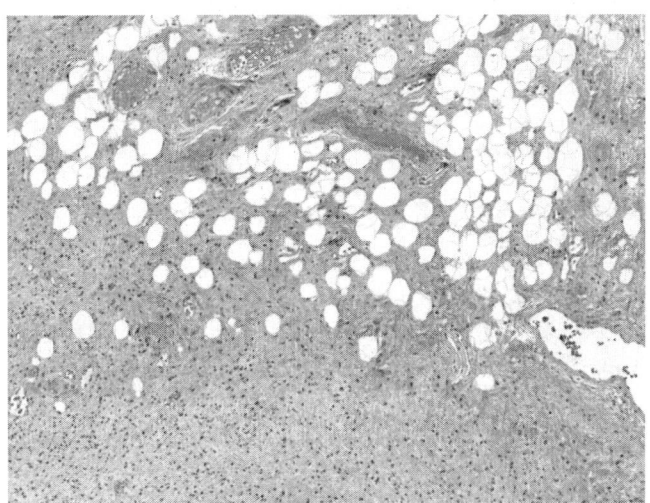

Figure 2. Neurofibroma diffusely growing and locally infiltrative into adipose tissue adjacent to the parotid gland (hematoxylin and eosin, original magnification 100X).

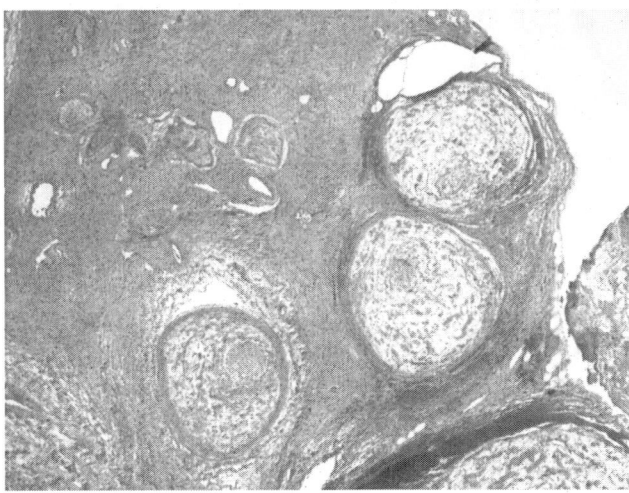

Figure 3. Plexiform neurofibroma marked by multiple nodules of neurofibromatous tissue (hematoxylin and eosin, original magnification 50X).

SCHWANNOMAS

Schwannoma is another benign tumor arising from peripheral nerve tissues from Schwann cells, as its name suggests. It has been previously referred to in the literature by other names such as neurilemoma and neurinoma. Schwannomas are thought to be associated with alterations or loss of the Neurofibromatosis type 2 (NF2) gene product (merlin), encoded for on chromosome 22 [15]. There is a well-known association of schwannomas with Neurofibromatosis type II and a rarer entity known as schwannomatosis [15, 16]. Prior radiation is also known to be a risk factor predisposing to the development of schwannoma [17]. About 9% of schwannomas arising from the facial nerve arise from the intraparotid segment [18]. Rare cases arising in the sublingual glands have been described [19].

The typical patient with an intraparotid schwannoma presents in the fifth or sixth decade of life with a slow growing, typically painless and mobile mass [20, 21]. A minority of cases may present with symptoms and signs related to facial nerve dysfunction, primarily secondary to compression of the nerve, or with pain [22, 23].

On imaging, as in other locations, the findings may be variable. Tumors are generally well circumscribed. On magnetic resonance imaging (MRI) studies, some tumors have been described as hyperintense on T1-weighted imaging with an enhancing peripheral rim on T2-weighted images; others lack this targetoid appearance [24, 25]. Cystic areas and areas of calcification may be seen. Bottom line, the imaging findings are not distinctive enough to allow distinction from other benign primary lesions of the salivary gland or other peripheral nerve sheath tumors.

Histologically, schwannomas in these locations look similar to schwannomas elsewhere. They are comprised of spindled cells with areas in which cells may be compactly arranged (Antoni A pattern) and other areas in which the cells are more rounded and more loosely arranged (Antoni B pattern) (Figures 4 and 5). Occasional tumors may have prominent numbers of macrophages or histiocytes in them, vascular sclerosis, hemosiderin deposition, cystic changes or myxoid change (Figures 6 and 7). A subset of tumors are marked by the presence of palisaded nuclei, referred to as Verocay bodies (Figure 8). Some tumors may demonstrate degenerative atypia marked by large hyperchromatic nuclei and smudgy chromatin pattern, referred to as "ancient change" [26]. Prominent mitotic activity is not a feature of schwannomas. Occasionally, focal necrosis may be evident. A subset of tumors are marked by prominent cellularity, so-called cellular schwannomas. A plexiform growth pattern has been rarely described in these tumors [27] and rarely epithelioid features may be evident. Melanotic schwannomas with psammoma bodies, associated with Carney complex and mutations of the PRKARIA tumor suppressor gene, have also been described [28, 29].

Immunohistochemistry-wise, schwannomas are characteristically uniformly positive with S-100 antibody. SOX10 immunostaining is also common. A minority of tumors may demonstrate patchy glial fibrillary acidic protein (GFAP) immunoreactivity. The capsule portion of the tumor may show scattered epithelial membrane antigen (EMA) positivity, due to the positive staining of perineurial cells.

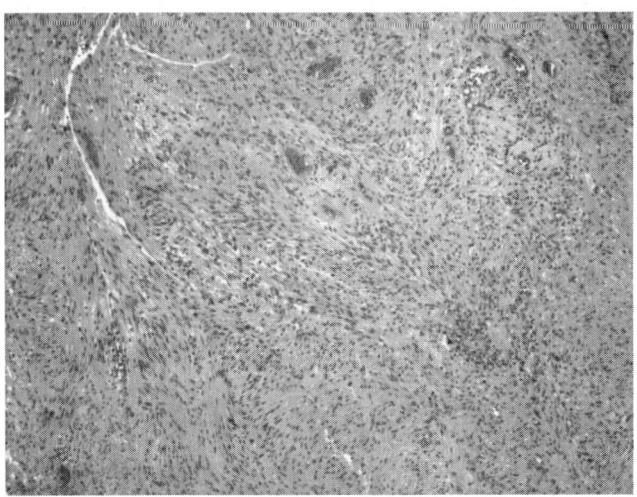

Figure 4. Schwannomas are marked by a proliferation of spindled cells. In areas such as seen here, the tumor cells are fairly tightly arranged, the so-called Antoni A pattern (hematoxylin and eosin, original magnification 100X).

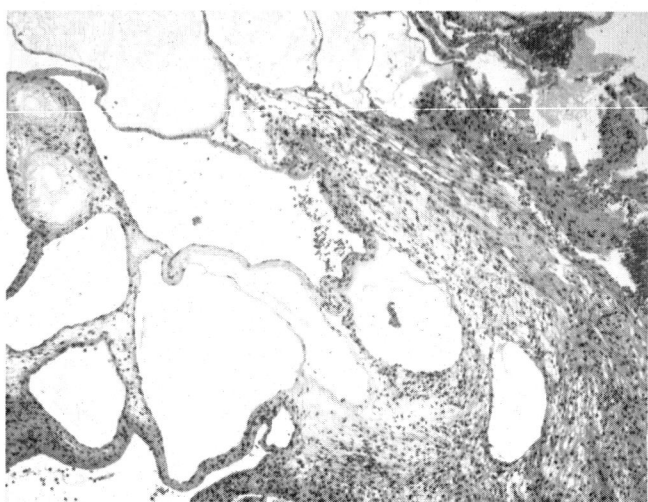

Figure 5. In other areas of a schwannoma, the cells are more loosely arranged and microcystic change may be present, the so-called Antoni B pattern (hematoxylin and eosin, original magnification 100X).

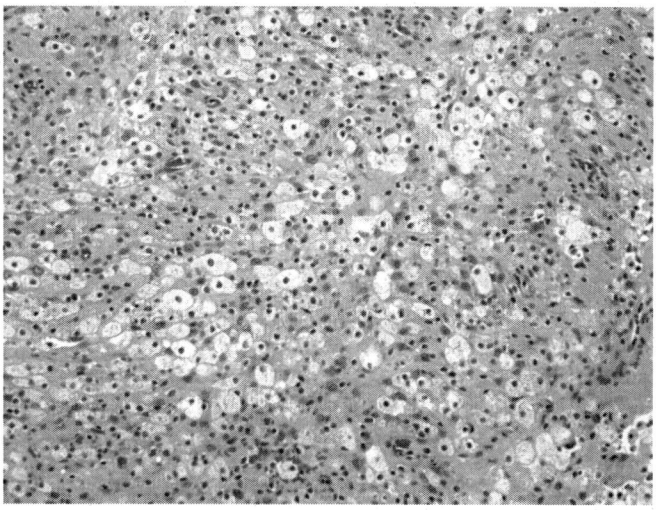

Figure 6. Macrophages, as seen here, may be focally prominently encountered in a schwannoma (hematoxylin and eosin, original magnification 200X).

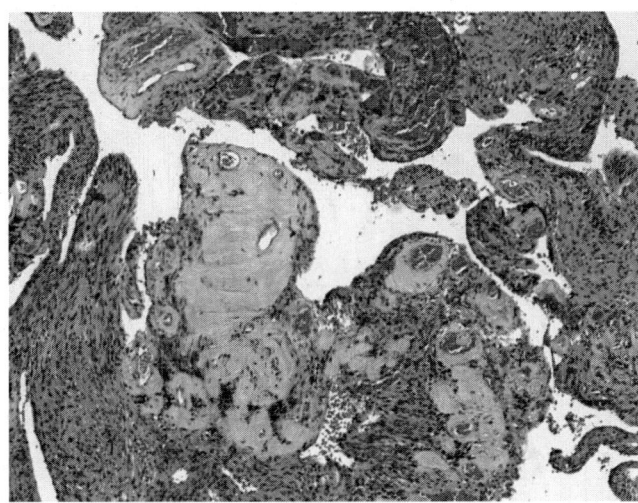

Figure 7. A schwannoma often shows prominent vascular sclerosis, as seen here. The tumor also shows hemosiderin deposition (brown pigment) and cystic changes (hematoxylin and eosin, original magnification 100X).

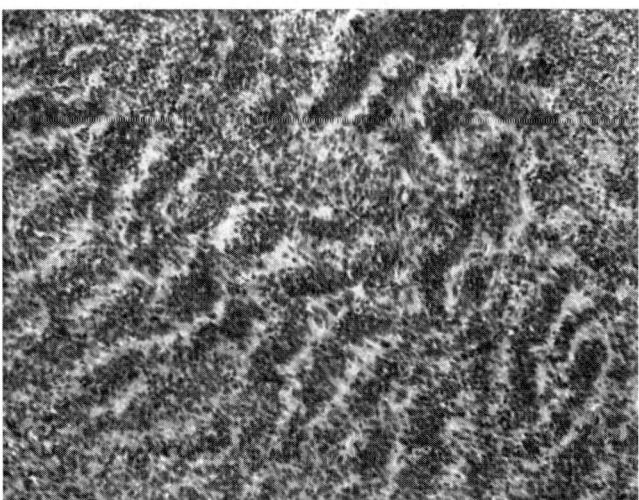

Figure 8. Another characteristic morphologic feature of some schwannomas in the presence of a palisaded pattern of tumor cell nuclei, known as Verocay bodies (hematoxylin and eosin, original magnification 200X).

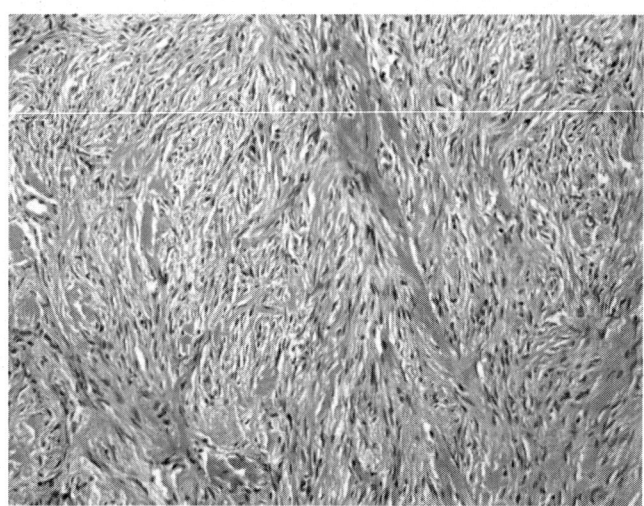

Figure 9. A solitary fibrous tumor can also arise in the salivary gland and is similarly marked by spindled cells. In contrast, collagen deposition is usually present between individual cells throughout the tumor. Solitary fibrous tumors also characteristically stain with antibody to STAT 6 (hematoxylin and eosin, original magnification 200X).

Differential diagnostic considerations include differentiating a schwannoma, particularly a tumor with a predominant Antoni B pattern, from a neurofibroma, a cellular schwannoma from a malignant peripheral nerve sheath tumor, a plexiform tumor from a plexiform neurofibroma, and a melanotic tumor from a melanoma. Neurofibromas, in contrast to schwannomas, are typically more ill-defined, nonencapsulated, uniformly hypocellular, and contain entrapped axons within the lesion (these can be highlighted with a neurofilament stain). Malignant peripheral nerve sheath tumors, as will be discussed shortly, are marked by increased mitotic activity. Solitary fibrous tumors arising in the salivary gland can also mimic the Antoni A pattern predominant schwannoma; solitary fibrous tumors are typically S-100 negative and stain with antibody to STAT 6 [30].

Management of intrasalivary gland schwannomas has been debated. Some believe conservative surveillance should be favored over surgical excision, especially in patients with minimal facial nerve dysfunction [20, 31]. With surgery also comes a risk of damaging or transecting the facial nerve. In the case of a patient who is symptomatic due to the tumor, an incisional biopsy to confirm diagnosis or excision, if there is a clear plane of resection between the tumor and facial nerve, is in order. If the facial nerve needs to be sacrificed to remove the tumor, a nerve graft may be employed, but this may come with some degree of permanent facial nerve dysfunction [20].

MALIGNANT PERIPHERAL NERVE SHEATH TUMORS (MPNST)

MPNSTs are malignant tumors arising from cells intrinsic to the nerve sheath. These tumors have previously been referred to by a variety of names in the literature including neurogenic sarcoma, neurofibrosarcoma and malignant schwannoma. The last of these terms is misleading, in that the vast majority of these tumors more typically either arise from neurofibromas that have undergone malignant degeneration or originate de novo from normal peripheral nerves and not schwannomas, which only rarely under malignant progression [32, 33]. Overall, MPNSTs comprise about 5% of all malignant soft tissue neoplasms and they are known to be associated with Neurofibromatosis type I in 50-60% of cases [34] and prior radiation [35].

Only rare cases of MPNST arising in the salivary glands have been documented in the literature [36-43]. Most arise in middle-aged adults; although tumors arising in the setting of Neurofibromatosis type I usually present at a younger age. These tumors typically present with signs and symptoms associated with a rapidly growing tumor, including pain and nerve palsy or dysfunction. Grossly, these are often larger masses which have a fleshy appearance due to the hypercellularity. Necrosis and hemorrhage are common findings. On imaging, the MPNSTs are characterized by irregular margins and heterogenous enhancement.

Microscopically, these tumors are characterized by hyperchromatic nuclei, increased cellularity, variable amounts of eosinophilic cytoplasm, and cytologic atypia (Figure 10). Increased mitotic activity is a common (Figure 11). Geographic areas of necrosis are frequently seen (Figure 12). Tumors may assume a variety of phenotypic appearances including that of a pleomorphic undifferentiated sarcoma. They may have an epithelioid appearance. Some tumors contain heterologous elements which may include an epithelioid component (such as glands or squamous epithelium) or mesenchymal component (such as cartilage or bone). Sometimes, a lower grade area resembling a benign neurofibroma or a normal appearing nerve or ganglion may be seen in association with the tumor.

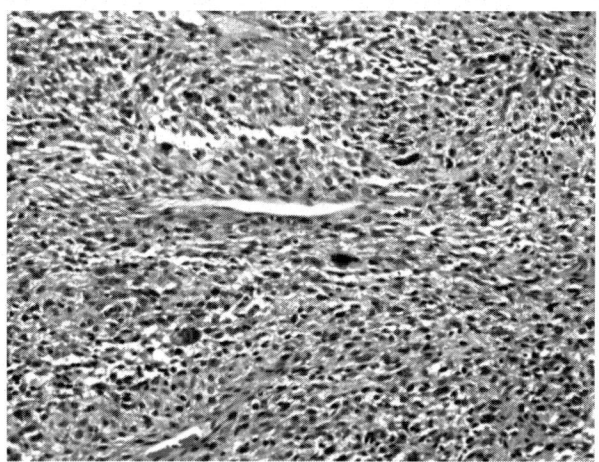

Figure 10. Malignant peripheral nerve sheath tumor of the parotid marked by prominent cellularity and nuclear atypia (hematoxylin and eosin, original magnification 200X).

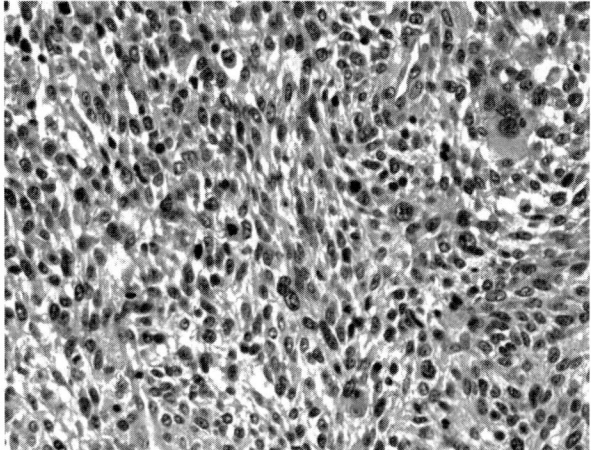

Figure 11. Mitotic figures are readily found in most malignant peripheral nerve sheath tumors (hematoxylin and eosin, original magnification 400X).

A subset of MPNSTs demonstrate S-100 immunoreactivity; the S-100 staining is more prominent in lower grade tumors and is more spotty in higher grade tumors. SOX10 positivity is observed in about half of tumors [43]. Heterologous elements will stain as expected with a host of other tissue specific markers. Low grade tumors may demonstrate some glial fibrillary acid protein (GFAP) immunoreactivity, which is typically absent in high grade tumors. Loss of H3K27me3 staining in tumor nuclei is also a fairly characteristic feature of these tumors, especially sporadic and post-radiation induced neoplasms [44].

From a genetic standpoint, MPNSTs are associated with NF1 gene inactivation, resulting in a loss of the neurofibromin protein, and TP53 mutations, which results in prominent p53 immunoreactivity in most tumors (not seen in neurofibromas) [45, 46]. p53 immunoreactivity, however, may be prominently observed in schwannomas. Deletion of the CDKN2A gene is also been noted in the majority of MPNSTs [45].

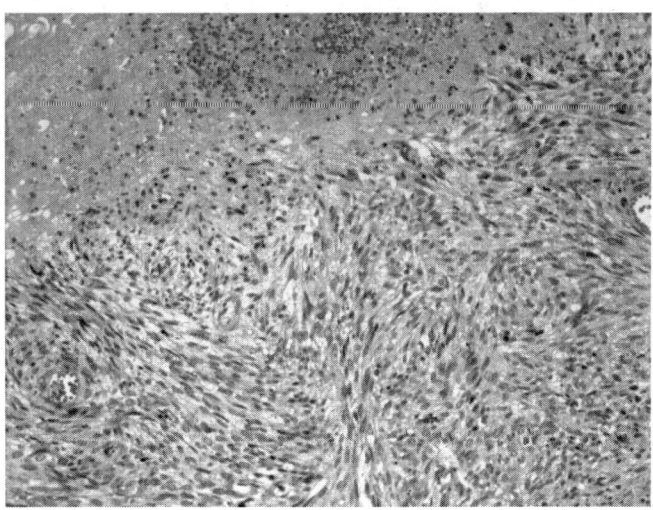

Figure 12. Geographic necrosis (top) is not an uncommon finding in malignant peripheral nerve sheath tumors (hematoxylin and eosin, original magnification 200X).

Wide excision of the tumor, to whatever extent that is possible is recommended; this may be challenging in the head and neck tumors. This may be accompanied by high dose radiation therapy or chemotherapy [36,

47]. Prognosis is generally poor, with 5 year survival of head and neck tumors being 23% in one series (in Neurofibromatosis type I patients) and 47% in patients without Neurofibromatosis type I [48]. Predictors of outcome in the head and neck based tumors included tumor size, location of the tumor and surgical margins [49]. Cases of tumors arising in the parotid gland and subsequently metastasizing to distant sites (skin, lung, bone and lymph node) have been documented [50].

REFERENCES

[1] Cho K-Y, Ro JY, Choi J, Choi S-H, Nam SYN, Kim SY. Mesenchymal neoplasms of the major salivary glands: clinicopathological features of 18 cases. *Eur. Arch. Otorhinolaryngol.* 2008; 265 (Suppl 1): S47-S56.

[2] Guraya SS, Prayson RA. Peripheral nerve sheath tumors arising in salivary glands: A clinicopathologic study. *Ann. Diagn. Pathol.* 2016; 23: 38-42.

[3] Woods D, Giguere C, Saliba L. Intraparotid neurofibroma: review of the literature. *J. Otolaryngol. Head Neck Surg.* 2001; 40: 104-112.

[4] Tati SY, Gole GN, Prabhala S, Gole SG. Plexiform neurofibroma of the submandibular salivary gland: a rare tumour. *Indian J. Surg.* 2011; 73: 224-226.

[5] Al Bisher H, Kant R, Aldamati A, Badar AA. Plexiform neurofibroma of the submandibular gland in patient with von Recklinghausen's disease. *Rare Tumors* 2011; 3E4:1012.

[6] Kosalka M, Miyanohara T, Mochizuki Y, Kamiishi H. A rare case of a facial nerve neurofibroma in the parotid gland. *Br. J. Plast. Surg.* 2002; 55: 689-191.

[7] Fadda MT, Verdino G, Mustazza MC, Bartoli D, Iannetti G. Intraparotid facial nerve multiple plexiform neurofibroma in patient with NF1. *Int. J. Pediatr. Otorhinolaryngol.* 2008; 72: 533-537.

[8] Qadri S, Rabindranath D, Khan AA, Senthil P. Neurofibroma arising in the parotid gland. A rare case report. *J. Med. Sci. Clin. Res.* 2016; 4(1): 88708874.

[9] Souaid J-P, Nguyen V-H, Zeltouni AG, Manoukian J. Intraparotid facial nerve solitary plexiform neurofibroma: a first paediatric case report. *Int. J. Pediatri. Otorhinolaryngol.* 2003; 67: 1113-1115.

[10] Rai A, Kumar A. Neurofibroma of facial nerve presenting as parotid mass. *J. Maxillofac. Oral. Surg.* 2015; 14(Suppl 1): S465-468.

[11] Martin N, Sterkers O, Mompoint D, Nahum H. Facial nerve neuromas: MR imaging – report of four cases. *Neuroradiology* 1992; 34: 62-67.

[12] Erlandson RA, Woodruff JM. Role of electron microscopy in the evaluation of soft tissue neoplasms, with emphasis on spindle cell and pleomorphic tumors. *Hum. Pathol.* 1998; 29: 1372-1381.

[13] Intraparotid facial nerve neurofibromas – McGuirt – 2009 – the laryngoscope – *Wiley online library* n.D. http://onlinelibrary.wiley.com/doi/10.1097/00005537-2003010000-00015/abstract [accessed June 10, 2019].

[14] Varan A, Sen B, Aydin B, Yalcin T, Kutluk T, Akyuz C. Neurofibromatosis type 1 and malignancy in childhood. *Clinical Genetics* 2016; 89(3): 341-345.

[15] Louis DN, Ramesh V, Gusella JF. Neuropathology and molecular genetics of neurofibromatosis type 2. *Am. J. Hum. Genet.* 1994; 55: 314-320.

[16] MacCollin M, Woodfin W, Kronn D, Short MP. Schwannomatosis: a clinical and pathologic study, *Neurology* 1996; 46: 1072-1079.

[17] Shore-Freedman E, Abrahams C, Recant W, Schneider AB. Neurilemomas and salivary gland tumors of the head and neck following childhood irradiation. *Cancer* 1983; 51: 159-163.

[18] Balle VH, Greisen O. Neurilemmoma of the facial nerve presenting as parotid tumors. *Ann Otol Rhinol Laryngol* 1984; 93(1): 70-72.

[19] Okada H, Tanaka S, Tajima H, Akimoto Y, Kaneda T, Yamamoto H. Schwannoma arising from the sublingual gland. *Ann. Diagn. Pathol.* 2013; 16(2): 141-144.

[20] McCarthy WA, Cox BL. Intraparotid schwannoma. *Arch. Pathol. Lab. Med.* 2014; 138: 982-985.
[21] Caughy RJ, May M, Schaitkin BM. Intraparotid facial nerve schwannoma: diagnosis and management. *Otolaryngol. Head Neck Surg.* 2004; 130(5): 586-592.
[22] Bretlau P, Melchiors H, Krogdahl A. Intraparotid neurilemmoma. *Acta Otolarngol.* 1983; 265(6): 699-703.
[23] Ma Q, Song H, Zhang AD, Hou R, Cheng X, Lei D. Diagnosis and management of intraparotid facial nerve schwannoma. *J. Craniomaxillofac. Surg.* 2010; 38(4): 271-273.
[24] Martin N, Sterkers O, Mompoint D, Nahum H. Facial nerve neuromas: MR imaging. *Neuroradiology* 1992; 34(1): 62-67.
[25] Suh J, Abenoza P, Galloway HR, Everson LI, Griffiths HJ. Peripheral (extracranial) nerve tumors: correlation of MR imaging and histologic findings. *Radiology* 1992; 183(2): 341-346.
[26] Ho C-F, Wu P-W, Lee T-J, Huang C-C. "Ancient" schwannoma of the submandibular gland. A case report and literature review. *Medicine* 2017; 96:51(e9134).
[27] dos Santos JN, Gurgel CAS, Ramos EAG, Junior FBP, Crusoe-Rebello IM, Oliveira MC. Plexiform schwannoma mimicking a salivary gland tumor: An unusual case report diagnosed in pediatric patient *Internal J. Pediatr. Otorhinololaryngol. Extra* 2011; 6: 317-321.
[28] Killeen RM, Davy CL, Bauserman SC. Melanocytic schwannoma. *Cancer* 1988; 62: 174-183.
[29] Stratakis CA, Kirschner LS, Carney JA. Clinical and molecular features of the Carney complex: diagnostic criteria and recommendations for patient evaluation. *J. Clin. Endocrinol. Metab.* 2001; 86(9): 4041-4046.
[30] Bauer JL, Miklos AZ, Thompson LDR. Parotid gland solitary fibrous tumor: A case report and clinicopathologic review of 22 cases from the literature. *Head Neck Pathol.* 2021; 6: 21-31.

[31] Gross BC, Carlson ML, Moore EJ, Driscoll CL, Olson KD. The intraparotid facial nerve schwannoma: a diagnostic and management conundrum. *Am. J. Otolaryngol.* 2012; 33(5): 497-504.

[32] Mikami Y, Hidaka T, Akisada T, Takemoto T, Irei I, Manabe T. Malignant peripheral nerve sheath tumor arising in benign ancient schwannoma; a case report with an immunohistochemical study. *Pathol. Int.* 2000; 50: 156-161.

[33] Woodruff JM, Selig AM, Crowley K, Allen PW. Schwannoma (neurilemoma) with malignant transformation. A rare, distinctive peripheral nerve tumor. *Am. J. Surg. Pathol.* 1994; 18: 882-895.

[34] Ducatman BS, Scheithauer BW, Piepgras DG, Reiman HM, Ilstrup DM. Malignant peripheral nerve sheath tumors. A clinicopathologic study of 120 cases. *Cancer* 1986; 57: 2006-2021.

[35] LaFemina J, Qin LX, Moraco NH, Antonescu CR, Fields RC, Crago AM, Brennan MF, Singer S. Oncologic outcomes of sporadic neurofibromatosis-associated, and radiation-induced malignant peripheral nerve sheath tumors. *Ann. Surg. Oncol.* 2013; 20(1): 66-72.

[36] Chis O, Albu S. Malignant peripheral nerve sheath tumor of the parotid gland. *J. Craniofac. Surg.* 2014; 25(5): e424-e426.

[37] Biswa P, Kar A, Mohanty L, Pattnaik K, Nayak M. Malignant peripheral nerve sheath tumor in parotid gland – A rare and challenging case. *J. Clin. Case Reports* 2013; 3(1): 1000243.

[38] Athow AC, Kirkham N. Malignant parotid salivary gland peripheral nerve sheath tumour in a twelve-year-old girl. *J. Larynol. Otol.* 1992; 106:748-750.

[39] Detafiano A, Kulamarva G, Citraro L, Borgia L, Corce A. Malignant peripheral nerve sheath tumour (malignant epithelioid schwannoma) of the parotid gland. *Bratisl. Lek. Listy* 2012; 113(10): 628-631.

[40] Punjabi AP, Haug RH, Chung-Park MJ, Likavek M. Malignant peripheral nerve sheath tumor of the parotid gland: report of case. *J. Oral Maxillofac. Surg.* 1996; 54: 765-769.

[41] Inamura S-I, Suzuki H, Usami S-I, Koda E, Yoshizawa A. Malignant peripheral nerve sheath tumor of the parotid gland. *Ann. Otol. Rhinol. Laryngol.* 2003; 112: 637-643.

[42] Nepka C, Karadana M, Karasavvidou F, Barbanis S, Kalodimos G, Koukoulis G. Fine needle aspiration cytology of a primary malignant peripheral nerve sheath tumor arising in the parotid gland: a case report. *Acta Cytol.* 2009; 53(4): 423-426.

[43] Gogate BP, Anand M, Deshmukh SD, Purandare SN. Malignant peripheral nerve sheath tumor of facial nerve: Presenting as parotid mass. *J. Oral. Maxillofac. Pathol.* 2013; 17(1): 129-131.

[44] Nonaka D, Chirboga L, Rubin BP. Sox10: a pan-schwannian and melanocytic marker. *Am. J. Surg. Pathol.* 2008; 32(9): 1291-1298.

[45] Prieto-Granada CN, Wiesner T, Messina JL, Jungbluth AA, Chi P, Antonescu CR. Loss of H3K27me3 expression is a highly sensitive marker for sporadic and radiation-induced MPNST. *Am. J. Surg. Pathol.* 2016; 40(4): 479-489.

[46] Lee W, Teckie S, Wiesner T, Ran L, Prieto Granada CN, Lin M, Zhu S, Cao Z, Liang Y, Sboner A, Tap WD, Fletcher JA, Huberman KH, Qin LX, Viale A, Singer S, Zheng D, Berger MF, Chen Y, Antonescu CR, Chi P. PRC2 is recurrently inactivated through EED or SUZ12 loss in malignant peripheral nerve sheath tumors. *Nat. Genet.* 2014; 46(11): 1227-1232.

[47] Halling KC, Scheithauer BW, Halling AC, Nascimento AG, Ziesmer SC, Roche PC, Wollan P . p53 expression in neurofibroma and malignant peripheral nerve sheath tumor. An immunohistochemical study of sporadic and NF-1 associated tumors. *Am. J. Clin. Pathol.* 1996; 106(3): 282-288.

[48] Wong WW, Hirose T, Scheithauer BW, Schild SE, Gunderson LL. Malignant peripheral nerve sheath tumor: analysis of treatment outcome. *Int. J. Radiat. Oncol. Biol. Phys.* 1998; 42: 351-360.

[49] Loree TR, North Jr JH, Werness BA, Nangia R, Mullins AP, Hicks Jr. WL. Malignant peripheral nerve sheath tumors of the head and neck: analysis of prognostic factors. *Otolaryngol. Head Neck Surg.* 2000; 122: 667-672.

[50] Colville RJI, Camilleri IG, McLean NR, Soames JV. Malignant peripheral nerve sheath tumour metastasizing to the parotid gland. *Br J Plastic Surg* 2003; 56(4): 418-420.

In: Nerve Sheath Tumors
Editor: Richard A. Prayson

ISBN: 978-1-53617-366-6
© 2020 Nova Science Publishers, Inc.

Chapter 5

MELANOTIC SCHWANNOMAS: A CLINICOPATHOLOGIC REVIEW

David Sin[1] and Richard A. Prayson[*], MD, MEd

Case Western Reserve University School of Medicine and Cleveland Clinic Department of Anatomic Pathology, Cleveland, Ohio, US

ABSTRACT

Melanotic schwannomas are relatively rare tumors of the peripheral nervous system. The tumor is well known to be associated with Carney's complex, an autosomal dominant hereditary tumor disorder, additionally marked by lentiginous pigmentation, Cushing's syndrome and myxomas of the heart, skin and breast. Tumors may present at any age and have been documented to arise throughout the body but with a predilection for the spinal nerves. Histopathologically, tumors are marked by spindled to epithelioid cells which contain neuromelanin pigment. A subset of tumors also show evidence of psammoma body formation. Although most tumors behave in a benign fashion, a subset of tumors, unlike conventional schwannoma, can follow a malignant course. Differential diagnostic considerations include other pigmented peripheral nerve sheath tumors,

---

[1] David Sin, BS.
[*] Corresponding Author's Email: praysor@ccf.org; Fax: 216-445-6967.

melanocytomas, melanomas, and clear cell sarcomas of soft tissue. This chapter will review the clinicopathologic features of these nerve sheath tumors including discussion of differential diagnosis.

INTRODUCTION

Melanotic schwannoma is a type of nerve sheath tumor also known as pigmented schwannoma, melanogenic schwannoma, and melanotic nerve sheath tumor [1–44]. These tumors are often circumscribed and comprised of melanin-producing cells. They typically exhibit ultrastructural features of Schwann cells. The majority of melanotic schwannomas are benign.

Melanotic schwannoma was initially described by Millar in 1932 as a pigmented tumor of a sympathetic ganglion [22]. The term "melanocytic schwannoma" for this condition was coined in 1975 by Fu et al. [23]. To date, there have been less than 200 cases of melanotic schwannoma [11]. Melanotic schwannoma represents less than 1% of all nerve sheath tumors [5].

CLINICAL PRESENTATION

The mean age of incidence for melanotic schwannoma is 38 years old, with age of diagnosis ranging from 10 to 84 years; there is no obvious gender predilection [5]. Melanotic schwannoma may occur throughout the peripheral nervous system but it often is found in the paraspinal sympathetic chain and gastrointestinal (GI) tract, in particular the esophagus and stomach [1–24, 26–43, 46]. The spinal nerves are affected by nonpsammomatous tumors more often, while the GI tract is more commonly affected by psammomatous tumors. Less frequent sites of involvement include the heart, liver, bronchus, trachea, soft tissues, bone, soft palate, cerebellum, orbit, cervix, and skin [5–8, 31, 32, 35, 38].

The symptoms of melanotic schwannoma are related to mass effect within an organ or soft tissue or nerve involvement. Thirteen percent of cases exhibit symptoms because of mass effect, while 35.5% of cases have symptoms suggesting nerve involvement [15]. Melanotic schwannoma may grow on bone, and such a case would present as pain and a bony mass [15, 35]. These tumors can also erode bone, and spinal nerve root tumors often cause expansion of vertebral foramina. Bone destruction is more often seen in malignant cases. Cutaneous melanotic schwannoma presents similarly to melanomas, and subcutaneous melanotic schwannoma resembles a slowly growing soft tissue mass [21]. Melanotic schwannoma may also be detected incidentally, as 29% of cases are asymptomatic [2].

Imaging can help with diagnosis and management of melanotic schwannoma [15, 36]. Radiographs and computed tomography (CT) often exhibit enlarged intervertebral foramina, bone erosion, and sclerosis in cases involving spinal nerves [15]. Melanotic schwannoma of the spine can be described as a soft-tissue tumor with a "dumbbell" morphology [15, 36]. Myelograms demonstrate the obstruction of contrast flow in the absence of spinal cord displacement [15]. Melanotic schwannomas contacting bone often shows sclerosis, cortical erosion, and local destruction.

Melanotic schwannoma presentation differs from that of conventional schwannomas in a variety of ways. For instance, melanotic schwannoma may recur locally and metastasize; whereas, conventional schwannomas do not [1, 2, 11]. Melanotic schwannoma primarily metastasizes to the lungs and pleura but may also travel to the pericardium, endocardium, mediastinum, diaphragm, bone, liver, and spleen [1, 2, 11, 15].

Fifty-five percent of patients with psammomatous melanotic schwannoma have Carney's complex, an autosomal dominant disorder [2]. The mean age of melanotic schwannoma diagnosis in patients with Carney's complex is 27 years, over 10 years earlier than for patients without Carney's complex. Carney's complex is characterized by the features of melanotic schwannoma in addition to lentiginous pigmentation; blue nevi; myxomas of the heart, skin, and breast; and endocrine overactivity involving the adrenal cortex, pituitary, testis, and thyroid [2, 24, 47]. Conventional schwannomas are not a feature of Carney's complex.

The lentiginous pigmentation of Carney's complex primarily involves the face (lacrimal caruncle, conjunctival semilunar fold, lips) and, in females, external genitalia. The blue nevi mainly affect a person's extremities and trunk, are usually multiple and small, and may be of the conventional or epithelioid type [24]. Endocrine overactivity associated with Carney's complex can cause Cushing's syndrome associated with pigmented nodular adrenocortical disease, acromegaly due to pituitary adenomas, and sexual precocity due to large cell Sertoli cell tumors of the testis.

GROSS FINDINGS

Melanotic schwannomas are multiple in a minority of cases [1, 2, 11, 41]. Most melanotic schwannoma lesions are at least 5 cm in diameter, circumscribed, and round to ovoid or sausage shaped. Melanotic schwannoma affecting spinal nerve roots are often dumbbell-shaped [2]. Large melanotic schwannoma lesions may be lobulated or cystic [2, 48, 49]. Melanotic schwannomas have a soft, firm, rubbery consistency although they may also be friable or hard [2, 14, 50]. Melanotic schwannoma lesions are enveloped by a thin connective tissue layer that can be interrupted by the infiltration of surrounding soft tissue, which is in contrast to the typically encapsulated conventional schwannoma [1, 2, 4]. These tumors are usually solid on a cut surface. They can display uniform or unevenly distributed tar black, blue, brown, or gray pigmentation. Some melanotic schwannomas display hemorrhage or necrosis [2, 14, 32, 48, 49]. Psammomatous melanotic schwannoma may show gross subcapsular calcification and metaplastic bone formation [2].

MICROSCOPIC FINDINGS

Most melanotic schwannoma lesions are highly cellular and are comprised of spindle-shaped and epithelioid cells. These cells are usually arranged in lobules, fascicles, or cellular whorls [1–11, 15, 17]. Features typical of conventional schwannomas, Verocay body-like structures, and microcyst formation are not common. The cells are also characterized by eosinophilic to amphophilic cytoplasm. The cells of melanotic schwannoma often display pink nuclear-cytoplasmic pseudoinclusions. They may also feature brown to black melanin granules deposited in variable amounts in the cytoplasm of spindle-shaped and epithelioid cells (Figure 1). The outlines of spindle cells may not be distinct in melanotic schwannoma but the cell borders of epithelioid cells are usually well-demarcated. Scattered multinucleated cells also are frequent in melanotic schwannoma. Infrequently, cells with vacuolated cytoplasm or clear cells are present [2]. Additionally, the nuclei of melanotic schwannoma cells are often round with delicate, evenly distributed chromatin and a small, distinct nucleolus (Figure 2).

Fontana-positive pigment obscures nuclear details in some instances of melanotic schwannoma. One can often see melanophages, or heavily pigmented macrophages, and small lymphocyte clusters in melanotic schwannoma. A potassium permanganate bleaching reaction for melanin may be needed to see the cytologic features of the pigmented cells (Figure 3) [51].

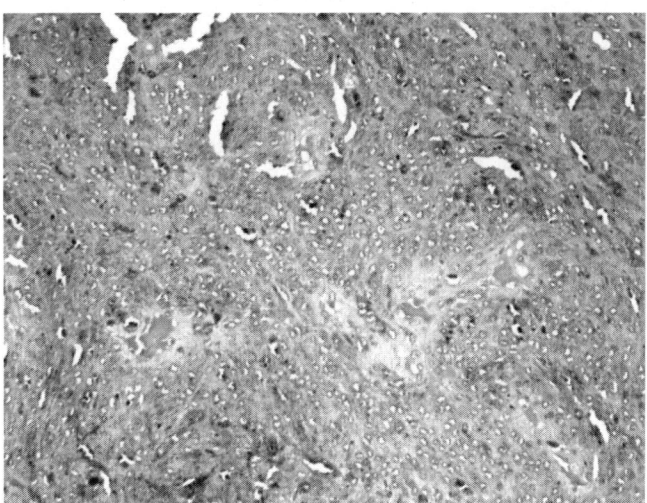

Figure 1. Melanotic schwannoma marked by epithelioid cells with increased brown melanin pigment in the cytoplasm (hematoxylin and eosin, original magnification 200X).

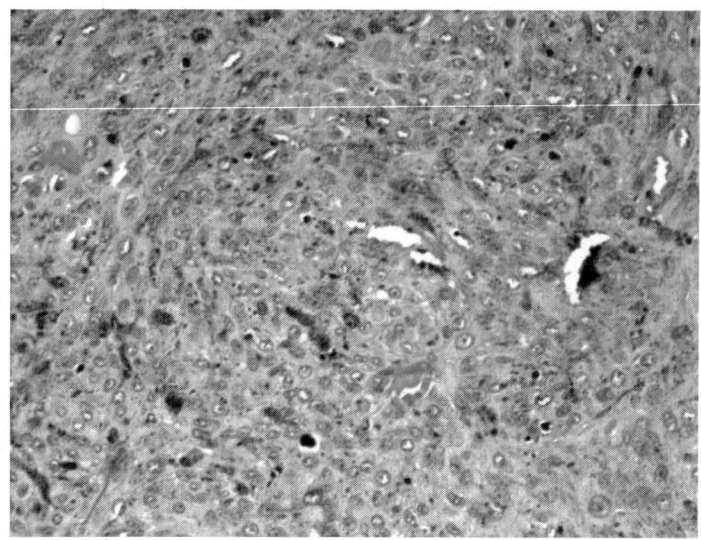

Figure 2. Prominent nucleoli are frequently observed in tumor cell nuclei (hematoxylin and eosin, original magnification 400X).

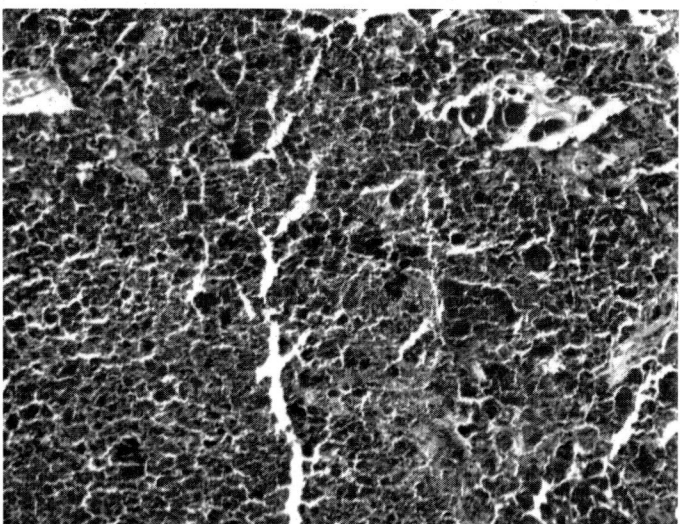

Figure 3. In some areas of the tumor, the amount of melanin pigment may be so prominent that it can be difficult to appreciate individual cell boundaries (hematoxylin and eosin, original magnification 200X).

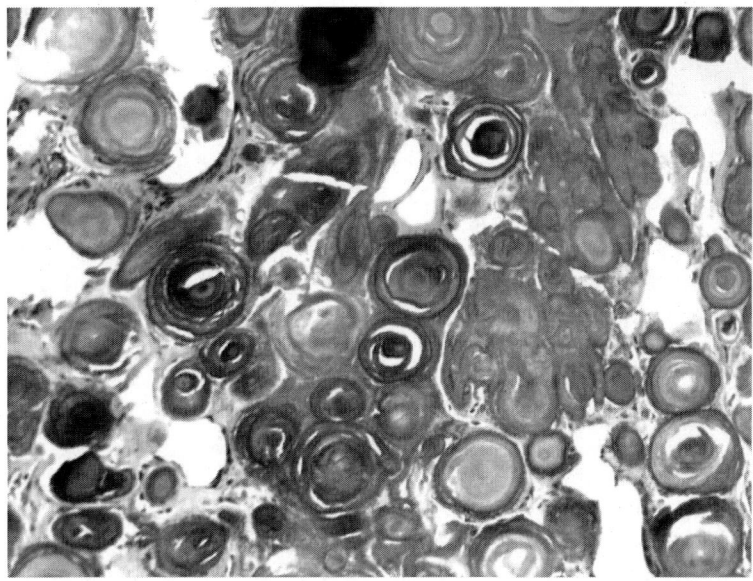

Figure 4. Occasional tumors may show calcifications and psammoma bodies (hematoxylin and eosin, original magnification 200X).

In melanotic schwannoma, an observer will rarely see only patches of pigmented cells. There may be myxoid change or stromal fibrosis. Psammomatous melanotic schwannoma specifically is characterized by laminated calcospherites in addition to the previously mentioned cytologic characteristics (Figure 4) [2]. Laminated calcospherites are PAS-positive spherical to oval, often focal, bodies. In melanotic schwannoma, vessels are thin-walled. This is in contrast to the thickened and hyalinized vessels of conventional sarcomas and many conventional schwannomas. Osseous metaplasia at the periphery of melanotic schwannoma is uncommon.

Malignancy may occur in melanotic schwannoma. If it does, it is usually associated with local recurrence. Clinically, malignant melanotic schwannomas have large, vesicular nuclei with scant chromatin and very prominent eosinophilic or violaceous macronucleoli. These malignant cells would also show increased mitotic activity, including abnormal mitoses, and broad zones of necrosis [11, 15].

IMMUNOHISTOCHEMICAL FINDINGS

The often bipolar, spindle-shaped, and epithelioid Schwann cells comprising benign and malignant melanotic schwannomas are immunoreactive for vimentin, S-100 protein, and HMB-45 [2, 32, 50, 52–55]. They are also positive for SOX10, Melan-A, p16, and the basement membrane markers laminin and collagen type 4 [1–11, 53]. So far, none have stained for glial fibrillary acidic protein (GFAP) [2].

ULTRASTRUCTURAL FINDINGS

Melanotic schwannoma can be characterized by clusters of spindle-shaped or plump cells with long, often interdigitating cytoplasmic processes. This description is mainly seen in the spinal nerves and sympathetic ganglia of melanotic schwannoma patients. Plump cells are joined together by occasional rudimentary cell junctions and free surfaces coated by a continuous and often reduplicated basement membrane. Melanosomes are notable in all stages of maturation in the cytoplasm of melanotic schwannoma cells [16, 17, 31, 32, 45, 50, 52–57]. Some nonspecific features of melanotic schwannoma include extracellular long-spacing collagen (Luse bodies), variable numbers of surface micropinocytotic vesicles, cytoplasmic intermediate filaments, and glycogen particles [16, 32, 45, 52].

GENETICS

The pathogenesis of melanotic schwannoma is poorly understood, and most melanotic schwannoma tumors are sporadic. Nevertheless, melanotic schwannoma often features a complex karyotype with recurrent monosomy of band 22q. It also may demonstrate variable whole chromosomal gains and recurrent losses, often of chromosomes 1 and 21 and chromosome arm 17p [58].

Fifty to 55% of psammomatous melanotic schwannoma cases are associated with Carney's complex. This autosomal-dominant condition is characterized by a mutation in chromosome 17 affecting *PRKAR1A*, which codes for the protein kinase cAMP-dependent type I regulatory subunit alpha [1–3, 10]. Two independent loci for Carney's complex have been found through genetic linkage analysis: CC1 located on bands 17p22-24 and CC2 located on band 2p16 [10]. The genetic defect at 2p16 that causes Carney's complex is unknown In most cases, Carney's complex is caused by inactivating mutations in the *PRKAR1A* gene located at 17q22-24 [10].

Psammomatous melanotic schwannoma can arise in neurofibromatosis type I (NF1) [33]. In contrast to the 17p22-24 *PRKAR1A* mutation associated with Carney's complex, NF1 features a mutated 17q11 band. Testing for *PRKAR1A* mutations is not recommended currently for patients with Carney's complex. However, such testing may be advised for detecting affected persons in families with known mutations of that gene to avoid unnecessary medical surveillance of noncarriers. Recent cytogenetic studies have showed trisomy 6p and ring chromosome 11 in melanotic schwannoma, suggesting that melanotic schwannoma may share some genetic abnormalities with malignant melanoma [44]. Of note, melanotic schwannomas lack a *BRAF* V600E mutation.

DIFFERENTIAL DIAGNOSIS

Melanotic schwannoma may present similarly to conventional schwannoma, pigmented neurofibroma, melanocytoma, metastatic melanoma, and clear cell sarcoma, but key differences do exist between these conditions. Distinguishing melanotic schwannoma from conventional schwannoma can be done readily. Melanotic schwannoma lacks a distinct capsule, well-formed Verocay bodies, and clear-cut Antoni A and B areas, all features of conventional schwannoma [1, 3]. Conventional schwannomas lack melanin, psammoma bodies, and fat; whereas, melanotic schwannomas possess these. Occasionally, lipofuscin in conventional schwannoma may resemble melanin, since it is a gray-brown granular pigment. Conventional schwannomas also rarely involve the GI tract while melanotic schwannoma is known to involve the GI tract commonly.

Differentiating melanotic schwannoma from a "pigmented neurofibroma" [59] and other pigmented peripheral nerve sheath tumors [59, 60] is more difficult. These neurofibromas are often of the diffuse type, varying in size, showing only microscopic pigment, and lacking psammoma bodies and fat [15, 59, 61–68]. The nuclei are small and often elongated in pigmented neurofibroma, while in melanotic schwannoma. The tumor cell may have a round nucleus with delicate chromatin and a distinct central nucleolus [3]. Melanotic schwannoma cells generally have abundant cytoplasm, while neurofibroma cells have scant cytoplasm. Immunostaining is not uniform in neurofibroma. The ultrastructural heterogeneity of cell types in neurofibroma contrasts with the uniform morphology of melanotic schwannoma cells.

Melanocytomas are CNS tumors showing mainly melanocytic features and can resemble melanotic schwannoma. Melanocytomas usually are found in the cranial or spinal leptomeninges [69–73], are usually demarcated, and compress their surroundings. Microscopically, they consist of heavily pigmented polygonal to somewhat elongate or occasionally dendritic cells with vesicular nuclei and prominent nucleoli [20, 74–77]. Mitoses are scant to absent in melanocytomas which are generally considered benign lesions [77]. Melanocytomas show similar hot-spot mutations in *GNAQ* and *GNA11* in codon 209 that resemble those in uveal melanomas and blue nevi [20, 77]. The melanocytoma immunoprofile is very similar to that of melanotic schwannoma, although staining for collagen type 4 is less abundant. A distinction may require electron microscopy. Both conditions share some features including variably pigmented melanosomes, occasional intermediate junctions, and basement membrane production. However, melanocytomas differ from melanotic schwannomas, since they lack psammoma bodies, adipose-like cells, pericellular basement membranes, and long-spacing collagen.

While metastatic melanoma and melanotic schwannoma can present similarly. Dendritic-appearing cells rarely appear in metastatic melanoma but are common in melanotic schwannoma. Melanomas rarely exhibit basement membrane formation and lack psammoma bodies and fat while melanotic schwannoma does characteristically show these features [3, 4, 78, 79]. Another distinguishing point between these conditions is the lack of the *BRAF V600E* marker in melanotic schwannoma contrasted with its presence in over 90% of melanomas [80–82].

Clear cell sarcoma, also known as soft tissue melanoma, may resemble melanotic schwannoma [83, 84]. It tends to invade soft tissues and grow micro- and macroscopically. However, the paucity or absence of pigment in its cells contrasts with the characteristic pigmentation of melanotic schwannoma. Similar to metastatic melanoma, clear cell sarcoma lacks psammoma bodies and fat and has not been shown to form basement membranes.

TREATMENT AND PROGNOSIS

Most cases of melanotic schwannoma are benign and slowly growing, although bone erosion may occur. Among those with malignant melanotic schwannoma, death due to disease, often by metastatic tumors, is equally frequent in non-psammomatous and psammomatous melanotic schwannomas. Some studies have shown that of all reported melanotic schwannoma patients, 15% of patients with non-psammomatous melanotic schwannoma and 15% of patients with psammomatous melanotic schwannoma died from their tumors [2, 23, 56, 85–88]. Melanotic schwannoma can present with multiple tumors, which makes differentiating primary and metastatic lesions challenging [2]. Some melanotic schwannoma patients with Carney's complex experience additional morbidity and mortality due to other associated conditions including endocrinopathy or cardiac myxomas [15]. The treatment of choice for primary melanotic schwannoma is surgical excision with tumor-free margins [5, 15].

CONCLUSION

Melanotic schwannomas are uncommon peripheral nervous system tumors. The tumor is associated with Carney's complex, an autosomal dominantly inherited tumor disorder characterized by lentiginous pigmentation and blue nevi, cardiac, cutaneous and breast myxomas, and endocrine hyperactivity. Tumors present at a mean age of 38 years with a tendency to involve the spinal nerves and GI tract. Histopathologically, tumors are marked by spindle-shaped to epithelioid cells that contain neuromelanin pigment. A subset of tumors also show evidence of psammoma body formation. Most melanotic schwannoma cases are benign, but some tumors, unlike conventional schwannoma, grow to become malignant. A differential diagnosis for melanotic schwannoma would include other pigmented peripheral nerve sheath tumors, melanocytomas, melanomas, and clear cell sarcomas of soft tissue. Surgical excision with tumor-free margins is the primary treatment.

REFERENCES

[1] Antonescu, C. R., Stratakis, C. A. Melanotic schwannoma. In: Fletcher CDM, Bridge JA, Hogendorn PCW, Martens F, editor. *Pathology and Genetics of Tumours of Soft Tissue and Bone*. IARC Press; 2013. p. 173.

[2] Carney, J. A. Psammomatous melanotic schwannoma. A distinctive, heritable tumor with special associations, including cardiac myxoma and the Cushing syndrome. *Am J Surg Pathol*. 1990;14: 206–222.

[3] Rodriguez, F. J., Stratakis C. A., Gareth Evans, D. Genetic predisposition to peripheral nerve neoplasia: diagnostic criteria and pathogenesis of neurofibromatoses, Carney complex, and related syndromes (Internet). *Acta Neuropathologica*. 2012. pp. 349–367. doi: 10.1007/s00401-011-0935-7.

[4] Kurtkaya-Yapicier, O., Scheithauer, B, Woodruff, J. M. The pathobiologic spectrum of schwannomas. *Histol Histopathol.* 2003; 18: 925–934.

[5] Gulati, H. K., Joshi, A. R., Anand. M., Deshmukh, S. D. Non psammomatous melanocytic schwannoma presenting as a subcutaneous nodule: A rare presentation of a rare lesion. *Asian J Neurosurg.* 2016;11: 317–318.

[6] Vallat-Decouvelaere, A. V., Wassef, M., Lot, G., Catala, M., Moussalam, M., Caruel, N., Mikol, J. Spinal melanotic schwannoma: a tumour with poor prognosis. *Histopathology.* 1999;35: 558–566.

[7] Li, B., Chen, Q. Melanotic schwannoma of thoracic spinal root mimics metastatic melanoma: a potential pitfall for misdiagnosis. *Int J Clin Exp Pathol.* 2015; 8: 8639–8641.

[8] Chetty, R., Vajpeyi, R., Penwick, J. L. Psammomatous melanotic schwannoma presenting as colonic polyps. *Virchows Arch.* 2007; 451: 717–720.

[9] Merat, R., Szalay-Quinodoz, I., Laffitte, E., Kaya, G. Psammomatous melanotic schwannoma: A challenging histological diagnosis. *Dermatopathology (Basel).* 2015; 2: 67–70.

[10] Rodriguez, F. J., Folpe, A. L., Giannini, C., Perry, A. Pathology of peripheral nerve sheath tumors: diagnostic overview and update on selected diagnostic problems. *Acta Neuropathol.* 2012; 123: 295–319.

[11] Torres-Mora, J., Dry, S., Li, X., Binder, S., Amin, M., Folpe, A. L. Malignant melanotic schwannian tumor: a clinicopathologic, immunohistochemical, and gene expression profiling study of 40 cases, with a proposal for the reclassification of "melanotic schwannoma." *Am J Surg Pathol.* 2014; 38: 94–105.

[12] Shields, L. B. E., Glassman, S. D., Raque, G. H., Shields, C. B. Malignant psammomatous melanotic schwannoma of the spine: A component of Carney complex. *Surg Neurol Int.* 2011;2: 136.

[13] Prieto-Rodríguez, M., Camañas-Sanz, A., Bas, T., Cortés, B., Vera-Sempere, F. J. Psammomatous melanotic schwannoma localized in the mediastinum: diagnosis by fine-needle aspiration cytology. *Diagn Cytopathol.* 1998; 19: 298–302.

[14] Killeen, R. M., Davy, C. L., Bauserman, S. C. Melanocytic schwannoma. *Cancer*. 1988; 62: 174–183.
[15] Siordia, J., Golden, T. Current discoveries and management of psammomatous melanotic schwannoma [Internet]. *J Cancer Tumor Internatl*. 2016. pp. 1–7. doi:10.9734/jcti/2016/23786.
[16] Mennemeyer, R. P., Hallman, K. O., Hammar, S. P., Raisis, J. E., Tytus, J. S., Bockus, D. Melanotic schwannoma. Clinical and ultrastructural studies of three cases with evidence of intracellular melanin synthesis. *Am J Surg Pathol*. 1979; 3: 3–10.
[17] Zhang, H., Yang, G., Chen, H., Wei, B., Ke, Q., Guo, H., Ye, L., Bu, H., Yang, K., Zhang, Y. H. Clinicopathological, immunohistochemical, and ultrastructural study of 13 cases of melanotic schwannoma. *Chin Med J*. 2005; 118: 1451–1461.
[18] Grayson, W., Hale, M. J. Epithelioid psammomatous melanotic schwannoma with osseous metaplasia. *Arch Pathol Lab Med*. 1998; 122: 285–287.
[19] Mees, S. T., Spieker, T., Eltze, E., Brockmann, J., Senninger, N., Bruewer, M. Intrathoracic psammomatous melanotic schwannoma associated with the Carney complex. *Ann Thorac Surg*. 2008; 86: 657–660.
[20] Küsters-Vandevelde, H. V., van Engen-van Grunsven, I. A., Küsters, B., van Dijk, M. R., Groenen, P. J., Wesseling, P., Blokx, W. A. M. Improved discrimination of melanotic schwannoma from melanocytic lesions by combined morphological and GNAQ mutational analysis. *Acta Neuropathol*. 2010; 120: 755–764.
[21] Kaehler, K. C., Russo, P. A., Katenkamp, D., Kreusch, T., Neuber, K., Schwarz, T., Hauschld, A. Melanocytic schwannoma of the cutaneous and subcutaneous tissues: three cases and a review of the literature. *Melanoma Res*. 2008; 18: 438–442.
[22] Millar, W. G., Gilbert Millar, W. A malignant melanotic tumour of ganglion cells arising from a thoracic sympathetic ganglion (Internet). *J Pathol Bacteriol*. 1932. pp. 351–357. doi: 10.1002/path.1700350305.

[23] Fu, Y. S., Kaye, G. I., Lattes, R. Primary malignant melanocytic tumors of the sympathetic ganglia, with an ultrastructural study of one. *Cancer.* 1975; 36: 2029–2041.

[24] Carney, J. A., Stratakis, C. A. Epithelioid blue nevus and psammomatous melanotic schwannoma: the unusual pigmented skin tumors of the Carney complex. *Semin Diagn Pathol.* 1998; 15: 216–224.

[25] Çulhaci, N., Dikicioğlu, E., Meteoğlu, I., Boylu, Ş. Multiple melanotic schwannoma (Internet). *Ann Diagn Pathol.* 2003. pp. 254–258. doi: 10.1016/s1092-9134(03)00073-x.

[26] Carney, J. A., Ferreiro, J. A. The epithelioid blue nevus. A multicentric familial tumor with important associations, including cardiac myxoma and psammomatous melanotic schwannoma. *Am J Surg Pathol.* 1996; 20: 259–272.

[27] Utiger, C. A., Headington, J. T. Psammomatous melanotic schwannoma. A new cutaneous marker for Carney's complex. *Arch Dermatol.* 1993; 129: 202–204.

[28] Martin-Reay, D. G., Shattuck, M. C., Guthrie, F. W., Jr. Psammomatous melanotic schwannoma: an additional component of Carney's complex. Report of a case. *Am J Clin Pathol.* 1991; 95: 484–489.

[29] Thornton, C. M., Handley, J., Bingham, E. A., Toner, P. G., Walsh, M. Y. Psammomatous melanotic schwannoma arising in the dermis in a patient with Carney's complex. *Histopathology.* 1992; 20: 71–73.

[30] Tawk, R. G., Tan, D., Mechtler, L., Fenstermaker, R. A. Melanotic schwannoma with drop metastases to the caudal spine and high expression of CD117 (c-kit). *J Neurooncol.* 2005; 71: 151–156.

[31] Font, R. L., Truong, L. D. Melanotic schwannoma of soft tissues. Electron-microscopic observations and review of literature. *Am J Surg Pathol.* 1984; 8: 129–138.

[32] Burns, D. K., Silva, F. G., Forde, K. A., Mount, P. M., Clark, H. B. Primary melanocytic schwannoma of the stomach. Evidence of dual melanocytic and schwannian differentiation in an extra-axial site in a patient without neurofibromatosis. *Cancer.* 1983; 52: 1432–1441.

[33] Murakami, T., Kiyosawa, T., Murata, S., Usui, K., Ohtsuki, M., Nakagawa, H., Malignant schwannoma with melanocytic differentiation arising in a patient with neurofibromatosis. *Br J Dermatol.* 2000; 143: 1078-1082.

[34] Carrasco, C. A., Rojas-Salazar, D., Chiorino, R., Venega, J. C., Wohlik, N. Melanotic nonpsammomatous trigeminal schwannoma as the first manifestation of Carney Complex [Internet]. *Neurosurgery.* 2006. pp. E1334–E1335. doi:10.1227/01.neu.0000245608.07570.d2.

[35] Kim, M., Choi, J., Khang, S., Kim, J., Lee, J., Cho, K. Primary intraosseous melanotic schwannoma of the fibula associated with the Carney complex. *Pathol Int.* 2006; 56: 538–542.

[36] Courcoutsakis, N. A., Tatsi, C., Patronas, N. J., Lee, C., Prassopoulos, P. K., Stratakis, C. A. The complex of myxomas, spotty skin pigmentation and endocrine overactivity (Carney complex): imaging findings with clinical and pathological correlation. *Insights Imaging.* 2013; 4: 119–133.

[37] Hilton, D. A., Hanemann, C. O. Schwannomas and their pathogenesis. *Brain Pathol.* 2014; 24: 205–220.

[38] Rowlands, D., Edwards, C., Collins, F. Malignant melanotic schwannoma of the bronchus. *J Clin Pathol.* 1987; 40: 1449–1455.

[39] Watson, J. C., Stratakis, C. A., Bryant-Greenwood, P. K., Koch, C. A., Kirschner, L. S., Nguyen, T., Carney, J. A., Oldfield, E. H. Neurosurgical implications of Carney complex. *J Neurosurg.* 2000; 92: 413–418.

[40] Steins, M. B., Serve, H., Zühlsdorf, M., Senninger, N., Semik, M., Berdel, W. E. Carboplatin/etoposide induces remission of metastasised malignant peripheral nerve tumours (malignant schwannoma) refractory to first-line therapy. *Oncol Rep.* 2002; 9: 627–630.

[41] Buhl, R., Barth, H., Hugo, H. H., Mautner, V. F., Mehdorn, H. M. Intracranial and spinal melanotic schwannoma in the same patient. *J Neurooncol.* 2004; 68: 249–254.

[42] Siordia, J. A. Medical and surgical management of Carney complex. *J Card Surg.* 2015; 30: 560–567.

[43] Claessens, N., Heymans, O., Arrese, J. E., Garcia, R., Oelbrandt, B., Piérard, G. E. Cutaneous psammomatous melanotic schwannoma: non-recurrence with surgical excision. *Am J Clin Dermatol.* 2003; 4: 799–802.

[44] Italiano, A., Michalak, S., Soulié, P., Peyron, A., Pedeutour, F. Trisomy 6p and ring chromosome 11 in a melanotic schwannoma suggest relation to malignant melanoma rather than conventional schwannoma (Internet). *Acta Neuropathol.* 2011. pp. 669–670. doi: 10.1007/s00401-011-0820-4.

[45] Krausz, T., Azzopardi, J. G., Pearse, E. Malignant melanoma of the sympathetic chain: with a consideration of pigmented nerve sheath tumours. *Histopathology.* 1984; 8: 881–894.

[46] Culhaci, N., Dikicioğlu, E., Meteoğlu, I., Boylu, S. Multiple melanotic schwannoma. *Ann Diagn Pathol.* 2003; 7: 254–258.

[47] Carney, J. A., Hruska, L. S., Beauchamp, G. D., Gordon, H. Dominant inheritance of the complex of myxomas, spotty pigmentation, and endocrine overactivity. *Mayo Clin Proc.* 1986; 61: 165–172.

[48] Christensen, C. Malignant melanocytic schwannoma. A case report. *Acta Chir Scand.* 1986; 152: 385–386.

[49] Theodossiou, A., Segditsas, T. (Intra-abdominally situated melanotic schwannoma). *Zentralbl Allg Pathol.* 1971; 114: 168–172.

[50] Erlandson, R. A. Melanotic schwannoma of spinal nerve origin. *Ultrastruct Pathol.* 1985; 9: 123–129.

[51] Sheehan, D. C. HBB, editor. Pigments and minerals. *Theory and practice of histotechnology.* 2nd ed. St. Louis: C. V. Mosby; 1980. pp. 214–232.

[52] Jensen, O. A, Bretlau, P. Melanotic schwannoma of the orbit. Immunohistochemical and ultrastructural study of a case and survey of the literature. *APMIS.* 1990; 98: 713–723.

[53] Miettinen, M. Melanotic schwannoma coexpression of vimentin and glial fibrillary acidic protein. *Ultrastruct Pathol.* 1987; 11: 39–46.

[54] Myers, J. L., Bernreuter, W., Dunham, W. Melanotic schwannoma. Clinicopathologic, immunohistochemical, and ultrastructural features of a rare primary bone tumor. *Am J Clin Pathol.* 1990;93: 424–429.

[55] Terzakis, J. A., Opher, E., Melamed, J., Santagada, E., Sloan, D. Intriguing Case: Pigmented melanocytie *schwannoma of the uterine cervix* (Internet). *Ultrastruct Pathol.* 1990. pp. 357–366. doi: 10.3109/01913129009032250.

[56] Janzer, R. C., Makek, M. Intraoral malignant melanotic schwannoma. Ultrastructural evidence for melanogenesis by Schwann's cells. *Arch Pathol Lab Med.* 1983;107: 298–301.

[57] Kayano, H., Katayama, I. Melanotic schwannoma arising in the sympathetic ganglion. *Hum Pathol.* 1988;19: 1355–1358.

[58] Koelsche, C., Hovestadt, V., Jones, D., Capper, D., Sturm, D., Sahm, F., Schrimpf, D., Adeberg, S., Bohmer, K., Hagenlocher, C., Mechtersheimer, G., Kohlhof, P., Muhleisen, H., Beschorner, R., Hartman, C., Braczynski, A. K., Mittelbronn, M., Buslei, R., Beckere, A., Grote, A., Urbach, H., Staszewski, O., Prinz, M., Hewer, E., Pfister, S. M., von Diemling, A., Reuss, D. E. Melanotic tumors of the nervous system are characterized by distinct mutational, chromosomal and epigenomic profiles. *Brain Pathol.* 2015;25: 202–208.

[59] Fetsch, J. F., Michal, M., Miettinen, M. Pigmented (melanotic) neurofibroma (Internet). *Am J Surg Pathol.* 2000. pp. 331–343. doi: 10.1097/00000478-200003000-00001.

[60] Payan, M. J., Gambarelli, D., Keller, P., Lachard, A., Garcin, M., Vigouroux, C., Toga, M. Melanotic neurofibroma: a case report with ultrastructural study. *Acta Neuropathol.* 1986;69: 148–152.

[61] Motoi, T., Ishida, T., Kawato, A., Motoi, N., Fukayama, M. Pigmented neurofibroma: review of Japanese patients with an analysis of melanogenesis demonstrating coexpression of c-met protooncogene and microphthalmia-associated transcription factor. *Hum Pathol.* 2005; 36: 871–877.

[62] Na, C. H., Song, I. G., Chung, B. S., Shin, B. S. Case of pigmented neurofibroma with hypertrichosis with no association to neurofibromatosis. *J Dermatol.* 2009;36: 541–544.

[63] Zhang, J., Jianmin, W. N. Pigmented neurofibroma in the superciliary arch (Internet). *Case Reports.* 2009. pp. bcr0820092140–bcr0820092140. doi: 10.1136/bcr.08.2009.2140.

[64] Inaba, M., Yamamoto, T., Minami, R., Ohbayashi, C., Hanioka, K. Pigmented neurofibroma: report of two cases and literature review. *Pathol Int.* 2001;51: 565–569.

[65] Novoa, R. A., Kovarik, C. L., Low, D. W., Argenyi, Z. Cutaneous epithelioid melanocytic neurofibroma arising in a patient with neurofibromatosis-1. *J Cutan Pathol.* 2014;41: 457–461.

[66] Pižem, J., Nicholson, K. M., Mraz, J., Prieto, V. G. Melanocytic differentiation is present in a significant proportion of nonpigmented diffuse neurofibromas: a potential diagnostic pitfall. *Am J Surg Pathol.* 2013; 37: 1182–1191.

[67] Ahn, S. K., Ahn, H. J., Kim, T., Hwang, S. M., Choi, E. H., Lee, S. H. Intratumoral fat in neurofibroma. *Am J Dermatopathol.* 2002; 24: 326–329.

[68] Val-Bernal, J. F., González-Vela, M. C. Cutaneous lipomatous neurofibroma: characterization and frequency. *J Cutan Pathol.* 2005; 32: 274–279.

[69] Brat, D. J., Giannini, C., Scheithauer, B. W., Burger, P. C. Primary melanocytic neoplasms of the central nervous systems. *Am J Surg Pathol.* 1999; 23: 745–754.

[70] Jellinger, K., Böck, F., Brenner, H. Meningeal melanocytoma. Report of a case and review of the literature. *Acta Neurochir.* 1988; 94: 78–87.

[71] Limas, C., Tio, F. O. Meningeal melanocytoma ("melanotic meningioma"). Its melanocytic origin as revealed by electron microscopy. *Cancer.* 1972;30: 1286–1294.

[72] Prabhu, S. S., Lynch, P. G., Keogh, A. J., Parekh, H. C. Intracranial meningeal melanocytoma: a report of two cases and a review of the literature. *Surg Neurol.* 1993;40: 516–521.

[73] Winston, K. R., Sotrel, A., Schnitt, S. J. Meningeal melanocytoma. Case report and review of the clinical and histological features. *J Neurosurg.* 1987;66: 50–57.

[74] Zembowicz, A., Carney, J. A., Mihm, M. C. Pigmented epithelioid melanocytoma: a low-grade melanocytic tumor with metastatic

potential indistinguishable from animal-type melanoma and epithelioid blue nevus. *Am J Surg Pathol.* 2004;28: 31–40.

[75] Zembowicz, A., Knoepp, S. M., Bei, T., Stergiopoulos, S., Eng, C., Mihm, M. C., et al. Loss of expression of protein kinase a regulatory subunit 1alpha in pigmented epithelioid melanocytoma but not in melanoma or other melanocytic lesions. *Am J Surg Pathol.* 2007; 31: 1764–1775.

[76] Marwaha, N., Batanian, J. R., Coppens, J. R., Pierson, M. J., Richards-Yutz, J., Ebrahimzadeh, J., Ganguly, A., Guzman, M. A. Subcutaneous melanocytoma mimicking a lipoma: a rare presentation of a rare neoplasm with histological, immunohistochemical, cytogenetic and molecular characterization. *J Cutan Pathol.* 2016;43: 1186–1196.

[77] Murali, R., Wiesner, T., Rosenblum, M. K., Bastian, B. C. GNAQ and GNA11 mutations in melanocytomas of the central nervous system. *Acta Neuropathol.* 2012;123: 457–459.

[78] DiMaio, S. M., Mackay, B., Smith, J. L., Jr, Dickersin, G. R. Neurosarcomatous transformation in malignant melanoma: an ultrastructural study. *Cancer.* 1982;50: 2345–2354.

[79] Prieto, V. G., Woodruff, J. M. Expression of basement membrane antigens in spindle cell melanoma. *J Cutan Pathol.* 1998;25: 297–300.

[80] Liu, W., Kelly, J. W., Trivett, M., Murray, W. K., Dowling, J. P., Wolfe, R., Mason, G., Magee, J., Angel, C., Dobrovic, A., McArthur, G. A. Distinct clinical and pathological features are associated with the BRAF(T1799A(V600E)) mutation in primary melanoma (Internet). *J Invest Dermatol.* 2007. pp. 900–905. doi: 10.1038/sj.jid. 5700632.

[81] Ritterhouse, L. L., Barletta, J. A. BRAF V600E mutation-specific antibody: A review. *Semin Diagn Pathol.* 2015;32: 400–408.

[82] Hodis, E., Watson, I. R., Kryukov, G. V., Arold, S. T., Imielinski, M., Theurillat, J. P., Nickerson, E., Auclair, D., Li, L., Place, C., Dicara, D. Ramos, A. H., Lawrence, M. S., Cibulskis, K., Sivachenko, A., Voet, D., Saksena, G., Stransky, N., Onofrio, R. C., Winckler, W., Ardlie, K., Wagle, N., Wargo, J., Chong, K., Morton, D. L., Stemke-Hale, K., Chen, G., Noble, M., Meyerson, M., Ladbury, J. E., Davies, M. A., Gershenwald, J. E., Wagner, S. N., Hoon, D. S., Schadendorf,

D., Lander, E. S., Gabriel, S. B., Getz, G., Garraway, L. A., Chin, L. A landscape of driver mutations in melanoma. *Cell*. 2012; 150: 251–263.

[83] Chung, E. B., Enzinger, F. M. Malignant melanoma of soft parts. A reassessment of clear cell sarcoma. *Am J Surg Pathol*. 1983; 7: 405–413.

[84] Enzinger, F, M. Clear-cell sarcoma of tendons and aponeuroses. An analysis of 21 cases. *Cancer*. 1965;18: 1163–1174.

[85] Cras, P., Ceuterick-de Groote, C., Van Vyve, M., Vercruyssen, A., Martin, J. J. Malignant pigmented spinal nerve root schwannoma metastasizing in the brain and viscera. *Clin Neuropathol*. 1990; 9: 290–294.

[86] Dastur, D. K., Sinh, G., Pandya, S. K. Melanotic tumor of the acoustic nerve (Internet). *J Neurosurg*. 1967. pp. 166–170. doi: 10.3171/jns.1967.27.2.0166.

[87] Graham, D. I., Paterson, A., McQueen, A., Milne, J. A., Urich, H. Melanotic tumours (blue naevi) of spinal nerve roots. *J Pathol*. 1976; 118: 83–89.

[88] Röyttä, M., Elfversson, J., Kalimo, H. Intraspinal pigmented schwannoma with malignant progression. *Acta Neurochir*. 1988; 95: 147–154.

EDITOR'S CONTACT INFORMATION

Richard A. Prayson, MD, MEd
Cleveland Clinic Lerner College of Medicine
of Case Western Reserve University
School of Medicine and Cleveland Clinic Department
of Anatomic Pathology
Cleveland Clinic Foundation
Cleveland, Ohio, US
Email: PRAYSOR@ccf.org

INDEX

A

acromegaly, 104
adjuvant chemotherapy, 16, 43, 68
adjuvant radiation, 43
Antoni A areas, 45
Antoni B areas, 45

B

blue nevi, 103, 110, 112
BRAF V600E, 17, 29, 38, 109, 111, 120
BRAF V600E mutations, 29, 38

C

calponin, 13
CD34, 24, 27, 45, 49, 52, 56, 58, 63, 67, 72
c-KIT, viii, 22, 24, 27, 30
claudin, viii, 22, 24, 26, 56, 58
claudin-1, viii, 22, 24, 26, 56
clear cell sarcoma, x, 101, 109, 111, 112, 121
collagen type IV, 25, 61
cytokeratin, 7, 13

D

desmin, 7, 24, 27, 30
diffuse neurofibroma, 50, 119
DOG1, 30

E

EMA, viii, 7, 13, 15, 22, 24, 27, 28, 29, 42, 49, 52, 56, 58, 59, 61, 63, 67, 72, 86, 89
endocrine overactivity, 103, 104, 116, 117
epidermal growth factor receptor, 16
epithelial membrane antigen, viii, 7, 22, 24, 27, 59, 86, 89
epithelioid malignant nerve sheath tumors, 2
epithelioid MPNST, viii, 1, 3, 4, 5, 6, 7, 8, 12, 14, 37
epithelioid sarcomas, 13
epithelioid schwannoma, 5, 9, 10, 15, 16, 18, 19, 99
EWSR1 gene rearrangement, 13
extraneural perineuriomas, 57

G

ganglioneuroma, 30
gastrointestinal stromal tumor, ix, 22, 30
GFAP, 7, 24, 45, 56, 63, 67, 89, 95, 108
gland, 85
glandular MPNST, 37
glial fibrillary acidic protein, 7, 24, 89, 108, 117
GLUT, 25, 56, 58
GLUT-1, 25, 56, 58
granular cell tumor, vii, ix, 35, 36, 38, 64, 66, 67

H

H3K27 trimethylation, 7, 18
hematogenous spread, 43

I

INI-1, 8, 11
intraneural perineuriomas, 22, 57, 58
irritation fibromas, 48, 49

K

Ki-67, 27, 42, 67

L

large cell Sertoli cell tumors of the testis, 104
laser ablation, 56
leiomyoma, ix, 22, 30, 66
lentiginous pigmentation, x, 101, 103, 112
LEOPARD syndrome, 66, 81
lipofuscin, 109
lockhern change, 55
luse bodies, 108
lysosomes, 66, 67

M

malignant, v, vii, viii, ix, x, 1, 2, 9, 11, 16, 17, 18, 19, 20, 23, 30, 35, 36, 37, 38, 40, 41, 42, 45, 47, 50, 53, 58, 61, 64, 65, 66, 67, 68, 69, 70, 71, 72, 78, 81, 82, 83, 84, 85, 87, 92, 93, 94, 95, 99, 100, 101, 103, 107, 108, 109, 111, 112, 113, 114, 115, 116, 117, 118, 120, 121
malignant melanoma, 2, 9, 11, 19, 109, 117, 120, 121
malignant peripheral nerve sheath tumor, vii, viii, ix, 1, 2, 16, 18, 19, 20, 36, 41, 42, 69, 70, 71, 72, 83, 84, 85, 92, 94, 95, 99, 100
malignant Triton tumor, 37
melan-A, 11
melanocytoma, 109, 110, 119, 120
melanosomes, 108, 110
melanotic schwannoma, x, 89, 101, 102, 103, 104, 105, 107, 108, 109, 110, 111, 112, 113, 114, 115, 116, 117, 118
metastatic melanoma, 19, 109, 110, 111, 113
metastatic poorly differentiated carcinoma, 15
MiTF, 63
MPNST with perineurial differentiation, 37
mucosal neuroma, vii, ix, 35, 36, 59, 60
multiple endocrine neoplasia type IIB, ix, 36, 60
myoepithelial carcinomas, 12, 13
myxomas, x, 101, 103, 111, 112, 116, 117

N

nerve, viii, ix, 1, 2, 16, 18, 20, 41, 42, 69, 70, 71, 72, 83, 92, 94, 99, 100

nerve sheath myxoma, vii, ix, 35, 36, 61, 62, 63
neurofibroma, vii, ix, 22, 30, 35, 36, 40, 50, 51, 52, 53, 56, 57, 74, 75, 76, 84, 85, 86, 87, 92, 94, 96, 97, 100, 110, 118, 119
neurofibromatosis type, ix, 2, 17, 18, 20, 23, 31, 32, 36, 37, 83, 85, 86, 87, 88, 93, 96, 97, 109
neurofibromatosis type 1/I, ix, 2, 18, 20, 23, 31, 32, 36, 37, 83, 85, 86, 87, 88, 93, 96, 97, 109
neurofibrosarcoma, 54, 76, 93
neurothekeomas, 61, 63
NF1 gene, 38, 39, 50, 95
NF2 gene, 43, 57
NKI/C3, 63

P

palisaded encapsulated neuroma, vii, ix, 35, 36, 54, 55
perineural invasion, 43
perineurial cells, viii, 21, 22, 23, 31, 36, 44, 50, 86, 89
perineurioma(s), v, vii, viii, ix, 21, 22, 23, 24, 26, 27, 28, 29, 30, 31, 32, 33, 35, 36, 56, 57, 58, 59, 77, 78
periodic acid-Schiff, 67
pigmented neurofibroma, 109, 110, 118, 119
pigmented nodular adrenocortical disease, 104
pigmented schwannoma, 102, 121
plexiform neurofibromas, ix, 39, 50, 51, 83
polyposis syndrome, 24
PRKAR1A, 109
psammomatous melanotic, 103, 104, 107, 109, 111, 112, 113, 114, 115, 117
pseudoepitheliomatous hyperplasia, 56, 65
PTPN11, 66, 81
pustule-ovoid bodies of Milian, 66

R

RAS signaling cascade, 38
RET proto-oncogene, 59

S

S-100 protein, viii, 7, 11, 22, 24, 27, 30, 31, 42, 45, 56, 58, 61, 63, 67, 86, 108
salivary gland tumors, 84, 85, 97
salivary glands, 84, 85, 93, 96
Schwann cells, 30, 31, 36, 43, 45, 47, 48, 50, 54, 55, 58, 85, 88, 102, 108
schwannoma, vii, ix, x, 3, 5, 9, 16, 17, 30, 35, 36, 43, 44, 45, 54, 56, 57, 64, 73, 74, 84, 88, 90, 91, 92, 93, 97, 98, 99, 101, 102, 103, 104, 105, 107, 108, 109, 110, 111, 112, 113, 114, 115, 116, 117, 118, 121
schwannoma have Carney's complex, 103
schwannomatosis, viii, 1, 43, 88, 97
SMA, 7, 13, 24, 27, 30
SMARCB1, viii, 1, 8, 9, 11, 13, 17, 18, 19
smooth muscle actin, 7, 13, 24, 27
soft tissue perineuriomas, viii, 21, 22, 26, 27, 28
solitary circumscribed neuromas, 54
SOX10, 45, 89, 95, 108
squamous cell carcinoma, 65
syndrome, x, 2, 60, 78, 101, 104, 112

T

traumatic neuroma, ix, 35, 36, 37, 47, 48, 49, 50, 54, 60

V

verocay, 31, 45, 46, 55, 56, 89, 91, 104, 109
verocay bodies, 31, 45, 55, 56, 89, 91, 109

vimentin, 24, 42, 56, 61, 63, 67, 86, 108, 117

W

Wagner Meissner bodies, 52, 53
Wallerian degeneration, 47, 48